fighting fatigue
and the Chronic Fatigue Syndrome

IAN BRIGHTHOPE

McCULLOCH POSITIVE HEALTH GUIDE

Allen & Unwin

Published 1991 by Allen & Unwin Pty Ltd
8 Napier Street, North Sydney, 2059

First published 1990 by McCulloch Publishing Pty Ltd
292 Rathdowne Street, North Carlton, Vic., 3054

Copyright © Ian Brighthope, 1990

Designed by Marius Foley
Typeset by Optima Typesetters, Brunswick, Vic.
Printed by The Book Printer, Maryborough, Vic.

Cataloguing-in-publication
Brighthope, Ian, 1946–
    Fighting fatigue and the chronic fatigue syndrome.
    ISBN 1 86373 157 1.
    1. Chronic fatigue syndrome. I. Title
616.8528

This book is copyright. Apart from any fair dealing for the purposes of private study, research, criticism or review as permitted under the Copyright Act, no part may be reproduced by any process without prior written permission from the publisher.

A McCulloch Positive Health Guide
produced for Allen & Unwin by
Susan McCulloch

Fighting Fatigue is not intended as medical advice. Its intent is solely informational and educational. Please consult the appropriate health professional should the need for one be indicated.

Contents

1. What is the chronic fatigue syndrome? 1
2. Depression 11
3. The causes of tiredness 29
4. Viruses, bacteria and candida 56
5. Chemicals, drugs and electro-magnetic radiation 75
6. Food and chemical sensitivity 106
7. Malnutrition in the chronic fatigue syndrome 120
8. Body pollution and detoxification 142
9. Mind power 181
10. An anti-fatigue management programme 194

References 218
Glossary 228
Index 233

To Jill

'The overuse of synthetic chemicals in agriculture, industry and medicine over the past few decades is the greatest uncontrolled experiment on humanity and life.'

Ian Brighthope

The Author

Ian Brighthope specialises in nutritional and environmental medicine, particularly in the treatment of the chronic fatigue syndrome, cancer, psychiatric disorders, heart disease, allergies, arthritis, skin diseases and asthma.

A graduate in both agricultural science and medicine, Ian Brighthope became interested in the implications of human nutrition and disease. His concern about the effects on the food chain of the increasing use of chemicals in agricultural production and food processing led him to investigate the consequences for the human nervous, immune and endocrine systems. Original research programmes are an integral part of his activities.

Dr Brighthope is president of the Australian College of Nutritional Medicine, a founding director of the Orthomolecular Medical Association of Australia, is a Fellow of both the International College of Applied Nutrition and the New York based Academy of Orthomolecular Psychiatry and is the principal lecturer for Australia's first post-graduate course in nutritional and environmental medicine which he pioneered. He lectures internationally to medical and health professionals and writes extensively for professional journals. His many publications include the books *The AIDS Fighters*, *You Can Knock Out Aids*, *Sleep Soundly Without Drugs* and *A Recipe for Health*.

CHAPTER ONE

What is the Chronic Fatigue Syndrome

Definition of fatigue

FATIGUE IS DEFINED as a weariness from bodily or mental exertion. It is usually a temporary reduction in the ability or functioning of the various organs, tissues, cells and other components of the body after excessive exertion or stimulation.

Fatigue is natural after vigorous exercise or a hard day's work. When it occurs at night prior to the usual sleeping time it is regarded as an accepted part of daily living.

Fatigue becomes a symptom of a more serious condition when it occurs more frequently and more severely than the usual tiredness that occurs at night. In fact, fatigue can be such a seriously debilitating symptom in many people that it has now become known as a disease in it's own right. This is called the chronic fatigue syndrome (CFS) which will be discussed in detail in later chapters.

Many people experience fatigue from time to time and can often pinpoint the reasons for their tiredness. It may be due to overwork, lack of sleep, extra stress in their life, poor diet, too much alcohol or unusual physical exertion. However, when this feeling of weariness, tiredness and exhaustion becomes too much and the ability or willingness to endure life and its day-to-day problems wanes, professional help should be sought to determine the exact causes of the fatigue and to receive appropriate treatment.

Consequences of the diminished ability to carry on day-to-day activities may include anxiety about the situation followed by depression. These symptoms are often complicated by fear, anger and resentment. A lack of harmony in interpersonal relationships often follows and may result in partnership separation, behaviourial problems especially in children, severe depression, alcoholism, drug dependence and sometimes even suicide.

The warning signs

Daytime fatigue and weariness is not a normal state. It appears that over the last two to three years, fatigue has become a more common symptom in the community. It has certainly been observed in the medical and healing professions as an increasing form of presentation for those seeking professional help.

Because fatigue can be a symptom of the early stages of many diseases, it should not be taken lightly. These diseases include serious medical conditions such as anaemia, heart disease, diabetes, allergies, psychiatric disorders including depression, auto-immune disease, respiratory disorders, chronic undiagnosed infection and stress.

A new disease called the chronic fatigue syndrome (CFS) should only be diagnosed after the others have been excluded. CFS has recently been defined by the orthodox medical profession. It is the severe fatigue which occurs after minimal muscle exertion and which persists for six months or longer. The actual cause of this chronic fatigue syndrome is not known but it is probably precipitated by one of a number of infectious agents, many of which are viruses, superimposed on a background of stress, poor nutrition and sensitivity to environmental pollutants.

It is interesting that many people who develop arthritis, heart disease, diabetes and even cancer say that they had been feeling tired, lethargic and without energy for some time prior to the onset of the full-blown disease. This period of time ranges from between six months and two years. Of course, with or without an end-stage disease low energy results in a life of dullness, apathy and depression.

It's not in the mind

A deficiency or lack of energy is not only physical but it can affect the mind and its basic mental functioning. This shows in a loss of concentration, poor short-term memory and a feeling of fuzziness in the brain or 'brain fag'. Many of these symptoms can be alleviated by determining the cause of the fatigue and treating it appropriately. For example, many women who suffer from the premenstrual syndrome (PMS or PMT) with irritability, anxiety, depression, fluid retention, breast tenderness and many other symptoms prior to the onset of their period, also suffer at that time from poor concentration and short-term memory problems. Many of these symptoms are the result of a deficiency in the activity of vitamin B6 and/or magnesium. Simply improving the diet and taking small to moderate doses of vitamin B6 and magnesium supplements may relieve or completely abolish these fatigue-associated symptoms.

Psychological stress and tension

Many people react adversely when confronted with a stressful situation. They may have actually 'learned' to be chronically stressed through habit. These people often develop increased muscular tension in stressful situations in readiness for activity. This increased muscle tension results in an overall contraction of the muscles throughout the body, including those of the head and neck, back, arms and lower limbs. As a consequence of this tension in the muscles, extra energy, nutrients and oxygen are utilised. Eventually, there is a build up of acids, including lactic acid and other waste products, in the over-utilised muscles. This results in tiredness and perhaps even muscular aches and pains.

If the stress and muscular tension persist for a long period of time, the result is migraine headaches, irritable bowel syndrome, joint pains, back pains, allergies, skin disorders and the whole complex range of psychosomatic disease.

The stress-tension-fatigue cycle can be vicious, but it can be stopped through stress management, diet, muscle stretching and exercise. It is important to attend to the psychological stress reactions which occur in life and to learn how to handle these situations adequately.

But in many individuals, fatigue itself can be a stress. The underlying cause of this stress fatigue must be determined before any psychological stress management techniques are useful.

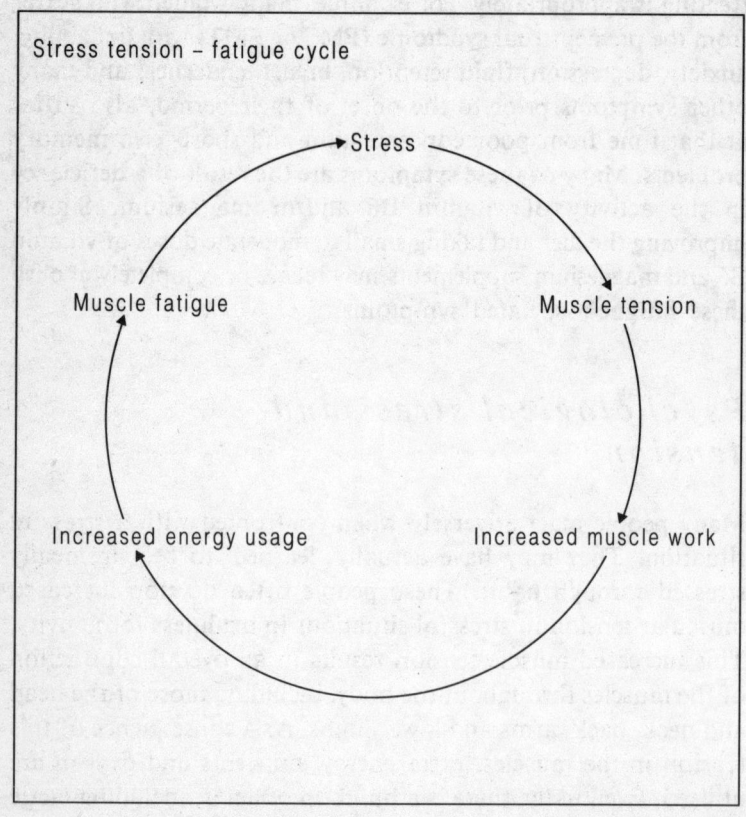

The chronic fatigue syndrome (post-viral fatigue syndrome or myalgic encephalitis)

The chronic fatigue syndrome (CFS) is another way of describing the extreme fatigue which may occur after an acute viral illness, influenza, a severe cold, hepatitis, glandular fever or gastro-enteritis. This syndrome includes severe fatigue which is the cardinal symptom, especially following minor exertion. Muscle aches and pains are also common. Difficulties with concentration, short-term memory loss, 'brain-fag' or fuzziness in the head, anxiety, depression, joint aches and pains, headaches, glandular swellings and fevers which are sometimes associated with sweats are not uncommon. Patients who have previously suffered with minor allergies tend to notice these allergies become worse. Individuals who never suffered from allergies discover to their amazement that they have become reactive to some foods and perhaps even chemicals in the environment.

Symptoms of CFS

1. Generalised fatigue
2. Impaired concentration
3. Difficulty with short-term memory
4. Muscle and joint pains
5. Headaches
6. Sleep disturbances
7. Difficulty in finding correct words
8. Irritability and emotional instability
9. Depression
10. Lymph node swellings

Sleep disturbances, and the inability to remain awake throughout the day, are common in this syndrome. In some people with the chronic fatigue syndrome a disorder very similar to narcolepsy develops. Narcolepsy is an uncontrollable desire to sleep and in some individuals may simply be a reflection of an underlying food or chemical sensitivity.

CFS generally affects young adults and it often occurs at times of increased stress. It is not uncommon for a teenager undergoing the rigours of competition during the final years of schooling to suffer sufficient stress and contract a glandular fever-like disease which bowls them over and may leave them an invalid for weeks, months and sometimes even years.

Younger children and older adults can also be affected. In all groups, the disease itself can cause months to years of severe suffering, not only as a consequence of extreme muscle fatigue and the other symptoms previously mentioned but also due to the associated nausea, indigestion, food and chemical sensitivities and the increased risk of infections and psychological problems which complicate the picture.

Because of the emphasis in modern medicine on diagnostic tests, doctors have, until recently, regarded this chronic fatigue as a psychological symptom of depression and have treated it as such. There are very few pathology tests readily available to the ordinary doctor which enable her or him to make a diagnosis of chronic fatigue syndrome. Many doctors and other health workers still believe that the chronic fatigue syndrome is 'all in the mind' and that 'you will just have to learn to live with it.'

However the disorder has actually been described in British medical literature since the 1930s. The earliest epidemic of CFS was in the Royal Free Hospital in London in 1955 when it was called the Royal Free Hospital disease. It has also been labelled 'Icelandic disease', 'Epidemic neurasthenia', 'Myalgic encephalomyelitis (ME)', 'Chronic fatigue syndrome' and the 'Post viral syndrome'. It was, and sometimes still is, inappropriately and unkindly referred to as the 'Yuppie flu'.

In Australia, more females than males appear to be affected by this disorder, particularly in the young professional groups. Young females tend to seek medical attention for the condition more often than males. If definite physical symptoms do not appear, males tend to withdraw from seeking further professional help. However, as time progresses the difference in apparent incidence of this disorder between the sexes is diminishing.

Myalgic encephalomyelitis (ME) — a non-diagnosis

Myalgic encephalomyelitis (ME) is a misnomer and a term which is probably best forgotten. The major symptom common to all these syndromes is muscle fatigue, and not muscle pain, which is suggested by the term myalgic. The major symptom of muscle fatigue after minor exertion may result in the inability to do anything at all for some time following that exertion. For example, walking from one end of a room to another may result in such severe fatigue that walking is impossible for another hour or two. Another example is that after reading a few lines of the newspaper, the muscles of the eyeballs become so fatigued that reading becomes impossible. Also, the term ME is inaccurate because encephalomyelitis suggests an inflammation of the brain and spinal cord. There is very little if any medical or scientific evidence for this. However, some health workers believe from indirect and clinical evidence that an allergic or immunological reaction is occurring in the central nervous system and this is responsible for causing many of the headaches, anxieties, depression, muscle weakness and other symptoms referrable to the nervous system.

It is interesting to note that recent scientific evidence has shown food allergens (proteins) can actually penetrate undigested across the small intestine into the bloodstream and pass via the blood to the brain and cross the blood-brain barrier, thus entering the nervous system. Foods may actually trigger immunological and other biochemical abnormalities in the central nervous system.

This helps to explain why some chronic psychiatric patients suffering schizophrenia, manic depression, psychotic depression and chronic anxiety respond very favourably to the withdrawal of known allergenic foods in their diet. Much more research work needs to be done in this area to provide us with an understanding of the underlying mechanisms and therefore a scientific approach to the management of these conditions.

History of ME and the chronic fatigue syndrome

A syndrome with fatigue being the major symptom has been recognised for over one hundred years. However, only recently has there been any serious research into this poorly understood disorder. Neurasthenia, which was believed to be a neurotic disorder associated with weakness and fatigue, was first described in 1880 by a Doctor George Beard. Outbreaks of the disorder were reported in Los Angeles in 1934, in Iceland in 1948 and in New York State in 1950.

The 1955 outbreak in the Royal Free Hospital in London involved more than 200 staff members, especially nurses. Surrounded by mystery, the Royal Free epidemic was later attributed to mass hysteria, and even today the psychiatric profession may in some cases confuse the condition with hysteria, depression or some weird anxiety state.

The triggers of fatigue

In the chronic fatigue syndrome, triggering factors quite often operate to bring on symptoms. These factors differ between and within individuals from time to time. For example, yeast, a very common allergen in bread, beer and wine may have no effect on a happy, contented individual during their annual vacations away from the smog of the city and the stress of everyday work. But on returning home even very small amounts of yeast may start triggering off allergic reactions again when the person is under more stress.

Most sufferers of chronic fatigue syndrome can pre-date their symptoms to an acute and/or severe viral infection. Others relate the onset of their disease to a bacterial infection involving the use of antibiotics. The inappropriate use of antibiotics without the consideration of a change in diet and the use of nutrient supplements to support immune function, may actually induce food and/or chemical sensitivities. Antibiotics are renowned for disturbing the growth of the normal micro-organisms and germs in the large intestine. In fact, the overgrowth of abnormal germs, yeast cells called candida (thrush) and pathogenic (disease-producing) bacteria in the large bowel, may be one of the most important sign-posts in directing the management of CFS. The acronym CFS not only represents chronic fatigue syndrome but also candida fungi spores and chemical food sensitivity — the relationships will be discussed in later chapters.

The bacteria, virus or germ that actually triggers CFS in one victim, may cause no more than a mild fever in other people. This is fairly strong evidence that the severity of the disease is determined by other factors, probably the most important being genetic individuality and the state of nourishment.

Probably the most important predisposing factor is the state of nutrition and the exposure to environmental pollutants at the time of the initial infection. Even a low level or mild deficiency of a single nutrient such as zinc, which is important for the proper functioning of the immune system, may leave an individual far more susceptible to a viral infection than an individual who is well nourished. There is extremely good evidence now that the Australian population does suffer from malnutrition with regard to one and quite often more than one specific nutrient.

In fact, our three major killer diseases — heart disease, cancer and stroke — have very strong nutritional factors in their causation. It is now believed by most responsible authorities that a change in diet can result in a reduction of the incidence of these three killers.

The chronic and persistent symptoms of CFS actually hint at profound disturbance of the two most sensitive systems of the body — the immune and nervous systems. From the evidence available it appears that the immune system does not seem to recover from the initial insult by the infective agent. Again, the unresolved nature of the disturbance of immune and nervous system functioning is probably determined by the state of nutrition and level of general pollution within the patient at the time of the initial viral assault. The nervous and immune systems go haywire as a consequence and find it difficult to return to normal activity, especially if they remain continually exposed to food and chemical sensitising agents, heavy metals, pesticide and herbicide residues and other highly oxidising compounds in the environment.

Controversial aspects

Ever since the term chronic fatigue syndrome has been coined there has been controversy. There has certainly been discussion within the medical profession itself about the actual name of the disease and some doctors still doubt its very existence.

Many people, both within the medical profession and the general community, still regard chronic fatigue with some scepticism. To them the answer to the question 'Is it a medical diagnosis, a psychiatric condition or the perfect description for a hypochondriac?' has yet to be provided.

However, more medical doctors and specialists are now regarding chronic fatigue syndrome as an organic disease with definite underlying pathology.

Social consequences

1. Labelled as malingerers
2. Repeated and inappropriate medical referrals
3. Medical over-treatment
4. Stigma of 'psychiatric' disorder
5. Poor employment record (often unemployable)
6. High dollar cost to the community
7. Divorce and separation
8. Alcoholism (or other addiction)
9. Suicide

Effective treatments for people with the chronic fatigue syndrome are available to prevent these dehumanising complications and even long-term sufferers can be helped. Some of the most successful results have occurred in the field of natural medicine where the therapist and patient can work together.

CHAPTER TWO

Depression — a mixture of fatigue and hopelessness

What is depression

DEPRESSION MEANS MANY things to many people. CFS-depression is the specific form of depression associated with the chronic fatigue syndrome. There is probably no satisfactory definition of pure depression because of the multitude of causes and possible methods of treatment. In simple terms, depression can mean being low in spirits or a reduction in vitality with feelings of sadness. Mild depression is seen largely as a loss of the usual pleasurable interests in the affairs of life, with a corresponding loss of spontaneity. Extra physical effort is required to perform normal everyday functions. Often the gratification and pleasure received in simple daily activities disappears.

Although a mildly depressed person does not necessarily have a severe physical illness, quite often they do suffer from symptoms of a physical nature including fatigue, lethargy, headaches, generalised aches and pains, constipation and loss of appetite — to mention a few. Often a depressed person will say that they feel neither well, relaxed nor comfortable in their normal surroundings. Lethargy, tiredness and fatigue are symptoms commonly complained about, and they often are excessive in nature. There is generally an increased awareness in ordinary bodily discomforts. Depressed people lose their positive feelings for life and such things as plans, hopes or goals become unimportant. Memories of the past are clouded and dull and bad memories, rather than good, are concentrated upon. Usually a person with mild depression can continue to do their daily chores, work, care for the family and function reasonably well in society. In fact, they may appear quite normal to most acquaintances. However, to their close friends and relatives the change to depression becomes obvious.

The appearance of a severely depressed person is unmistakable. They look dejected and unhappy, lack joy and a sense of humour and have a general 'down in the dumps' attitude. There is usually an associated severe loss of self-esteem. In a depressed person a sense of hopelessness prevails and they are usually unresponsive to any attempt at a rational discussion. A general slowing down of physical activity, including speech and movement, may be obvious. Thinking may also be slowed down, resulting in a slowing of mental processes and mental efficiency which can affect work and relationships. An anxious, restless, agitated and tense depressed person finds it difficult both to be alone and to be in the company of others.

This tension and depression is often felt by other people in the presence of a depressed person. The depressed individual with associated anxiety is usually the complainer. They can be a 'painful person'. They suffer unnecessary guilt. Feelings of unworthiness, lethargy, apathy, hopelessness, gloom and doom, black moods and aches and pains prevail. In the severest forms of depression, the patient may actually have complicated false beliefs about him or herself to the point where they may imagine that they have a severe disease such as cancer. A change for the worse in sleeping habits, which often become severe and disturbing, is probably the most common of the problems experienced by a depressed person. They often find it difficult to get to sleep or remain asleep. Restless nights in bed are very common. Consequently, fatigue and lethargy become more pronounced and further aggravate the depression.

Early morning wakening is a common problem for a severely

depressed person. They usually wake with the blues and without an eagerness to start the day. It is this wakefulness with fatigue in the early hours of the morning which creates more disgust for life and even deep misery. Occasionally increased sleeping patterns occur in depression and these may, or may not, be associated with alcohol or drug abuse. Weight loss and a loss of appetite also occur in depression. In fact, the reduced intake of healthy food in a person who has a loss of appetite will further aggravate depression. Depressive people also complain of other physical symptoms including abdominal pains, bloating, constipation, occasional wind, premenstrual depression, tension, further tension, breast tenderness, irregular periods, headaches, generalised aches and pains and as mentioned before, severe fatigue.

Another classical symptom of depression is a loss of interest in sex or a reduction in capacity of sexual activity. In fact, the four basic animal appetites are reduced in depression i.e. the loss of appetite for food, activity, sex and sleep.

Depression is a very painful thing. It can be lethal. Depression is a very common disorder in our community and it is increasing. At the tip of the iceberg, we find that 33% and 25% of women and men respectively seek help from a doctor for depression in her/his lifetime. For some, that lifetime is shortened. Despite great advances in medicine generally and some advances in psychiatric treatments, depression is still a killer. Beneath the tip of that iceberg is a growing base problem of depression in the general community. Left untreated, its cost to society is incalculable. CFS-depression is no exception.

Anne's story

'I didn't know what it was like to feel well,' was Anne's response after 25 years of drug and shock treatment every four to six months for chronic depression.

Anne had suffered from a debilitating flu-like illness for over three weeks that did not respond to the usual bed rest, antibiotics and aspirin; in fact, she actually deteriorated while taking these drugs. She never completely recovered from this illness and suffered from many non-specific symptoms including tiredness, muscle weakness, headaches, abdominal pains, premenstrual tension and backache for years afterwards.

The advice of many doctors and specialists was sought but nothing organically wrong could be found. Finally, a psychiatrist diagnosed depression and she was given medication for her nerves. Within two weeks of taking this medication she became irrational, severely depressed and suicidal. It was decided to hospitalise her; more medications were prescribed which depressed her even more, resulting in a suicide attempt. Electric shock treatment was given and after eight courses of this her depression lifted. Shock treatment can be life-saving in severe cases such as Anne's but today there are better ways of treating and preventing depression.

Unfortunately, the relief Anne experienced was short-lived and for the next 25 years she received drugs and shock treatment. Eventually, on the advice of a friend, she decided to seek an alternative opinion because she still suffered greatly from debilitating fatigue.

A young neurologist diagnosed her as suffering from myalgic encephalomyelitis, a controversial disease. Anne had heard of a doctor who was successfully treating many ME patients by changing their diet and giving them large doses of vitamins and other nutrients both orally and by injection.

Anne deteriorated after commencing this treatment and became extremely agitated and angry. This was the first time in 20 years that she had felt such anger and she blamed her new doctor and his injections for her state. It took a couple of minutes of questioning before she realised that with the onset of her anger had come an incredible amount of energy and an almost miraculous lifting of her depressed mood.

Once Anne realised what was happening and she was given a naturally occurring herbal tranquilliser to help calm down her newly-activated nervous system, her recovery from decades of illness was final. Anne is now helping to run the family business and is busy doing fund-raising and looking after grandchildren — activities that she was never able to undertake. Anne's diagnosis has also been changed to the chronic fatigue syndrome caused by chemical sensitivity and aggravated by a vitamin dependency state. A vitamin dependency state occurs sometimes as a consequence of chronic stress. Many prisoners of war, for example, starved in concentration camps need to take high doses of certain B group vitamins to stay well. In Anne's case, her 'stresses' were chemical drugs, electric shock treatments and 'depression'.

The causes of depression

There is no single cause of depression. If there was, the treatment would be relatively simple. However, this is generally not the case, particularly with people who have had depression for a long time and have become severely depressed, with consequent changes in both their physical and personality traits.

But we may consider a large number of factors which contribute to, or aggravate, a person's mood changes. Mood swings are normal in all of us. These swings are usually gentle, from the feeling of well-being where very little bothers us to sometimes feeling gloomy and sad, but still knowing that there is light at the end of the tunnel. These minor mood swings are a normal part of life. It is when the swings become severe that we must pay attention to them. Someone heading for the pits of depression needs help. That help can come in many forms and by paying attention to some of those 'causes', or factors contributing to depression, we can help prevent that downhill slide. Many of the causes of depression overlap with the causes of chronic fatigue syndrome and in any one patient, a major single factor may be involved in making a major contribution to both states.

Causes of depression

A. Genetic (inherited) factors
B. Nutritional factors

C. Social factors
D. Environmental factors
E. Medical and psychological factors
F. Drug and substance abuse factors

A. Genetic (inherited) factors

Depression tends to occur more commonly in some families than in others. Considering the importance of neurotransmitters in brain function and the fact that their activity is dependent on diet and enzyme function, the role of gene-dependent enzyme activity is obvious. No case of depression is purely due to inherited or environmental factors.

B. Nutritional factors

i.   Food and chemical sensitivities
ii. Functional reactive hypoglycaemia (low blood sugar)
iii. Nutritional deficiencies and imbalances
iv. High sugar consumption or sugar hypersensitivity
v.   Chronic candidiasis with sensitivity to yeasts and thrush

C. Social factors

i.   Relationships, e.g. family problems, problems with partner or children.
ii. Losses, e.g. loss of loved one, loss of status/self-esteem, loss of an object — burglary, house fire, threatened or imagined losses
iii. Unemployment
iv. Bereavement
v.   Lifestyle changes, e.g. shifting home, changing jobs, inability to spend time on recreational activities

D. Environmental factors

i. Weather changes
ii. Lunar cycles, e.g. full moon

iii. Environmental chemicals and synthetics
iv. Electromagnetic radiation
v. 'Sick building' syndrome
vi. Jetlag
vii. Poor work environment, e.g. polluted air, noise, difficulties with colleagues, etc.
viii. Poor home environment, e.g. arguments with partner, overcrowding, different values, etc.

E. Medical and psychological factors

i. Chronic pain syndrome
ii. Other chronic illnesses
iii. Chronic abnormal stress reaction
iv. Specific hormone changes e.g. during adolescence, menstruation, childbirth, menopause

F. Drugs and substance abuse factors

i. Alcohol and tobacco
ii. Caffeine
iii. Illicit drugs (e.g. marijuana and heroin)
iv. Medically prescribed drugs including opiate based pain killers, blood pressure drugs, beta-blockers, cortisone, oral contraceptive pill, tranquillisers, sedatives, antihistamines, anti-epileptic medications.

Depression — a chemical imbalance

Since ancient times depression has been a recognised illness. But as we can see from the above list of factors contributing to depression, it should be better regarded as a mixture of different disorders. At the top of the list of causative factors we should perhaps list genetic and inherited factors. Severe depression appears to be more common in some families than others. When we consider that the brain and nervous system, which may be the seat of nervous and depressive disorders, is a complex mixture of chemicals that are in part dependent on our food intake and in part on our inherited ability through enzymes to change this chemical composition, depression becomes more logical. Even Sigmund Freud stated that neuroses and mental disorders were probably chemical imbalances which would one day be discovered. Psychiatrists can use drugs to alter a few chemical imbalances in the brain and nutritionists can use food and nutritional supplements to do the same, more safely.

Effects of a depressive illness

The most horrifying effect of depression is suicide. A person who is threatening suicide or who indicates that life is not worth living should immediately seek psychiatric treatment.

Fortunately, most people who suffer from depression realise that sooner or later their illness will subside and their feelings of sadness, hopelessness, guilt and many of the physical symptoms will improve. An attack of depression which comes on suddenly usually lasts from a few days up to about six months, depending of course on the severity of the attack and on the treatment given. In the more severe forms of depression which are associated with mental illness, the depression is more likely to be recurring. In a few very unfortunate patients, repeated attacks may result in a severe mental disorder or even schizophrenia.

In the majority of people, depression usually results in the lowering of moods and the feeling of hopelessness at work, home and play. A slowing of the thinking processes, including the inability to concentrate and make important decisions, affects their everyday life. There is a loss of interest and a reduction in their involvement in work and family and social activities. Without the usual sexual drive, the relationship between partners can often be strained in depression to the point of separation and divorce.

Excessive sleep, or the inability to sleep, certainly has an effect on the household. The depressed person waking in the middle of the night, watching TV in the early hours of the morning or raiding the refrigerator, may be disturbing to the rest of the family. These aberrations of behaviour cause anxieties and tensions within the family which distress everybody and result in further disturbed relationships.

Not only is there a slowing in the thinking processes in the depressed person, but he or she may also suffer from a slowing down of physical activities. They may find it difficult to become motivated to do things around the house or at work and may sit idly in a chair for long periods of time. False beliefs about their own health and self-esteem occur and minor aches, pains and physical symptoms, which most of us overlook, become major problems. A depressed person often appears to be a hypochondriac. As a consequence of many of these problems, delusions occur and the person may suffer from unusual fears and therefore withdraw from social activities.

Some physical symptoms which occur as a result of depression are loss of appetite and weight loss. This loss of appetite may be caused by a reduction in the appreciation of food which often occurs as a result of nutritional deficiencies. For example, a deficiency of zinc in the diet can result in a loss of the sense of taste and smell. Low zinc also causes depression, apathy, lethargy and anorexia. These zinc deficiency problems further aggravate the person's depression. Consequently, they tend to eat less and become more and more deficient in more and more nutrients — nutrients especially important in the functioning of the nervous system and brain.

It has been very well documented scientifically that the majority of patients entering a psychiatric or mental institution have multiple deficiencies of a wide range of nutrients and micronutrients. This low intake of nutrients is a compounding factor in the downhill spiral to the depths of depression.

Depression is a reality of everyday life and is something we can learn to deal with — sometimes very easily and very simply.

Diagnosis — how is it made?

The depressed person can often partly understand their depression and self-diagnosis is possible. However, a moderately depressed individual suffering from a whole range of symptoms associated with depression may not recognise the illness. When a person understands that he or she is feeling dejected and despondent, with feelings of hopelessness and sadness, and they can talk freely about these feelings, then the diagnosis can be easily made by a qualified doctor or psychologist.

If a person's symptoms are mainly physical and include such things as fatigue, lethargy, headaches, poor sleep, reduced sex drive, aches and pains, loss of weight and loss of appetite, then the diagnosis is not so easily made.

If the depression is severe enough, with delusions of a persecutory nature, and the individual is withdrawn, then the uncommunicative attitude which tends to occur in these people makes the diagnosis even more difficult.

Often people with an underlying depression will simply complain about chronic fatigue. This seems to be their major symptom and yet when questioned in depth other physical symptoms become obvious. In such cases, where the predominance of symptoms are physical in nature and the depression is of a secondary degree, the person's problems are more than likely physical and not purely psychological or psychiatric. In fact, most patients with depression and physical symptoms are found to be suffering from food chemical sensitivity aggravated by low levels of essential nutrients for the brain and nervous system including amino acids, trace elements, minerals and vitamins.

A depressing life event occurring before the onset of a depressive type of illness does add weight to the psychological and social nature of depression. However, that depressing life event may have been simply a stress factor sufficient to disturb a shaky biochemistry and push it into the malfunction mode. For example, if a person has been functioning quite well but not eating adequately, and drinking more alcohol than they should, a stressful life event can increase the body's utilisation of certain nutrients. If these are not replaced sufficiently, and within a certain time, the system becomes deficient in these nutrients and will start to malfunction.

Quite often these depressing life events are clear to family and friends but not to the depressed person. This is where expert psychiatric and medical check-ups are essential to rule out any physical causes for symptoms prior to the diagnosis of depression being made as a purely psychiatric or psychological phenomenon. In fact, if we consider the list of causes and associated factors in depression it becomes clear that the disorder is simply a word

— a description of a feeling — and not a true disease. It is a descriptive term for the way an individual feels and as such should be cautiously applied.

It is important to remember that the identification of a life stress event, or the presence of mental symptoms in a depressed person, is not sufficient evidence to exclude a physical disease or biochemical imbalance. A very severe depression in which the patient is totally non-communicative may be due to a severe medical disorder or a severe psychiatric illness (psychosis). These are obvious problems that should be immediately attended to medically and/or psychiatrically.

In the severely depressed person it must be emphasised that the depression may be a symptom occurring as a consequence of some other psychiatric disorder. This requires psychiatric and medical evaluation in order to differentiate between the different forms of depression. If the depression is associated with a severe psychiatric disorder or psychosis it is usually necessary to hospitalise the patient for immediate treatment to reduce the risk of suicide. In the very severe forms of depression such as this, the ability to concentrate and remember events are severely affected. The sufferer is usually riddled with feelings of guilt and false beliefs. Early morning wakening and weight loss are prominent symptoms. The greatest risk of suicide in a depressed person occurs when they are tense and agitated. An inability to relax, pacing the floor, wringing the hands and an overall bodily restlessness are indications requiring immediate attention and hospitalisation.

Another very often confusing symptom is that of masked depression — the person who appears with a big smile — the smiling depressive. Often it doesn't take long to break through the barrier in these depressed people to discover a sudden onset of weepiness and an almost shattered individual pouring out their heart with problem after problem. But before reaching this stage it is often very difficult, because of compensating mechanisms, to find a mood disturbance. Often it is a simple triggering factor, such as the mention of the death of a loved one or the separation of a spouse, which suddenly substitutes the smiling joyful facade with gloom, doom and buckets of tears.

Abnormalities in behaviour such as are seen in people with obsessions regarding work, sex or cleanliness, may also be a substitute for a defence against some forms of depression.

Symptoms of depression (most common to CFS)

Feelings of sadness and hopelessness
Low moods
Feelings of guilt and anger
Inability to concentrate
Reduction in memory
Difficulty thinking
Inability to make decisions
Loss of interest in work, play, family and friends
Reduced sleep
Excessive sleep
Disturbed sleep (often occurs long before depression)
Tension and anxiety
Reduced interest in sex and sexual activities
Slowing down of physical and mental activities
Hypochondriacal symptoms
Almost total withdrawal from life's activities (severe depression)
Loss of appetite and weight
Severe insomnia (severe depression)
Substance abuse e.g. drugs, alcohol, tobacco (especially a recent increase in use)
Obsession with suicide
Suicide attempts

Types of depression

It is important to distinguish between the various types of depression because the more severe forms can result in suicide. Also, some of the most severe forms of depression require expert medical and psychiatric assessment and treatment.

But most patients with mild to moderate depression and fatigue can, with the aid of the suggestions in this book, help themselves to better mental and physical health. There are many fancy classifications of depression and none of them are very satisfactory.

Mild to moderate depression

These forms of depression occur as a result of some adverse situation occurring in a person's life, such as the loss of a person by death, separation, divorce or loss of employment or financial independence. Associated with these losses are feelings of anger and resentment which, if not expressed, result in feelings of guilt. Usually based in this group of mild to moderate depression are symptoms of a milder nature ranging from feelings of sadness, hopelessness, worry, poor concentration, anxiety and a loss of interest in everyday activities. The loss of energy and associated functions in the chronic fatigue syndrome cause further depression.

Major depression without obvious outside cause

This severe form of depression occurs relatively independently of a person's lifestyle and life situation or events. It is sometimes called endogenous depression. There may be a significantly higher incidence of the chronic fatigue syndrome occurring in subpopulations of endogenous depressives. Complaints of course are more severe than in the mild to moderate forms of depression and include a loss of interest in life's activities and loss of pleasure in living, associated with the withdrawal from activities such as work, play and other social events. The consequences of this withdrawal are feelings of guilt and sometimes anger. Symptoms of poor memory, the inability to concentrate, tension, anxiety, chronic lethargy and fatigue, feelings of worthlessness and a loss of interest in sex are also common. Complaints of a physical nature which may be regarded as psychosomatic are also common and include headaches, backaches, abdominal pains and general 'unwellness'. In this group of people suffering depression, variations in symptoms occur, usually with symptoms being more severe in the mornings and gradual improvement occurring as the day progresses.

Disturbances of sleep are very common in the more severe forms of depression, particularly early morning wakening. A loss of appetite and weight loss, often associated with abdominal pain and constipation, are common. People with severe depression may suffer from tension and agitation and this is usually an indication for hospitalisation and psychiatric care. False beliefs about themselves and others may also exist and they may also suffer from irrational fears and thoughts. They may be very suspicious about other people and their ideas. They may have false beliefs that minor bodily symptoms are indicative of such things as a heart attack, ulcer or even cancer.

Occasionally, a person with severe depression may have mood changes in the opposite direction, including a feeling of extreme well-being, elation, sometimes an over-involvement in general life activities. Feelings that they can accomplish anything are common and they may believe that they have very little need for sleep. This is known as a mania, and when it is associated with swings of mood to depression it is called manic-depression. The person in a manic episode is usually very over-active and over-enthusiastic about everything and their unusual behaviour may range from doing the housework at 2a.m. to excessive financial commitments, making hasty decisions about major issues such as employment or marriage or even exhibitionist behaviour. Generally these episodes of mania are of shorter duration than the episodes of depression and the mania may be combined with irritability, aggressive behaviour and unstable moods which can result in disastrous consequences with relationships.

Depression secondary to other diseases

Any illness or disease can result in a mild, moderate or even severe depression. Simple viruses such as a cold, flu or even glandular fever may cause depression in some people. If the symptoms are severe and debilitating, the interference with a person's life and activities may be profound. Significant depression generally occurs with more severe conditions such as chronic heart disease, debilitating asthma and emphysema, rheumatoid arthritis and severe degenerative disorders like multiple sclerosis, Parkinson's disease, dementia and diabetes with all of its complications.

Severe mental diseases such as schizophrenia may from time to time be associated with moderate to severe depression. Alcohol and medical drugs, such as blood pressure pills, beta-blockers, corticosteroids, the oral contraceptive pill, tranquillisers, sedatives, opium-based pain-killing drugs and antihistamines, can also cause depression.

Risk of suicide

Suicide is the major complication of any depressive illness and the risk of suicide increases the longer the duration of the chronic fatigue syndrome.

The longer depression or a depressive illness exists, the more it becomes crystallised as a part of the personality. Over time the personality becomes more and more negative, and when life is no longer worth living and there is no sense of hope, the risk is very real. Some suicide attempts are performed in the presence of another person, with the prime object of controlling or doing some sort of injury to that other person.

Many suicide attempts are made by people who feel totally overwhelmed by their everyday problems in living. Most people who attempt suicide for this reason often don't really want to die but cannot see any way of continuing as they previously had been. People with severe depression may not attempt suicide whilst in that state. However, when the depression lifts and they commence to improve they may make a serious attempt on their life at this stage. It is therefore important for severe depressives to be cared for in hospital while being treated, because as their depression lifts their levels of activity increase. It may be just a sufficient increase in level of activity for them to overcome the inertia and perform the self-destructive act.

With severely mentally disturbed people, suicide attempts are often unpredictable and very successful.

It is very important to recognise the tense, anxious, agitated, depressed individual with a severe mental illness because it is just this person who is likely to jump off a building or shoot him/herself.

The painful patient

A chronic illness or disease of any kind may contribute to depression. It may even be the prime cause for depression, particularly if the disorder is associated with pain of any nature; chronic pain can make anyone depressed at times. However, quite often the reverse is true and a patient with depression will complain of vague aches and pains, sometimes constantly, from head to toe. In such a patient it is very important to look for substances in the person's environment, such as food allergies, chemical sensitivities or the overuse of substances such as coffee, tea, chocolate, cola, sugar or alcohol. Certain foods including dairy products, cereal grains and members of the nightshade family (potatoes, tomatoes, capsicums, tobacco and eggplant) may aggravate 'pain syndromes'. All of these may contribute to, or aggravate, fatigue and depression in a sensitive individual.

The chronic fatigue syndrome (the post-viral fatigue syndrome or M.E. — myalgic encephalomyelitis

This is simply another way of describing extreme fatigue following an acute viral illness such as influenza, glandular fever or even hepatitis. The cardinal symptom is severe muscle fatigue especially following minor exertion. This may simply be the inability to move due to fatigue after walking from one side of a room to another. Or it may reflect itself in the inability to read anything more than a couple of lines of the newspaper before the eye muscles give in. Other symptoms of this syndrome include muscle aches and pains, difficulties with concentration and memory, depression, anxiety, headaches and swelling of the glands.

The longer the condition persists, the greater the problems with psychological and psychiatric disorders including depression. In fact, the depression can become so severe that thoughts of suicide occur. In individuals with the chronic fatigue syndrome there is also a high rate of divorce and separation and a greater incidence of alcoholism.

Despite the lack of effective medical help for people with this problem, there are ways of treating them. The earlier they are treated the better the outcome and the quicker the response to therapy.

One important point that must be made here is that the whole issue of a depressive illness is confused by the very fact that the word is used as an expression of a disease, a symptom or a mood. It must be recognised that there are many factors contributing to depressive illness and that usually more than two of these factors play major contributing roles to the progression of the condition.

By addressing the many causes and aggravating factors

simultaneously, or as much as possible, a far more effective clinical outcome can be achieved. In fact, by adopting the dietary lifestyle approaches to the management of depression, millions of people world-wide have already been helped either to reduce the severity, frequency or duration of attacks. To quote one patient — 'This is the best I have felt in thirty years — in fact I never knew what it felt like to be well'.

Easy relief, without drugs, from mild to moderate depression

The simplest and sometimes the most effective way of relieving mild to moderate depression is to make simple changes to your lifestyle, habits and diet.

There is increasing medical and scientific information to show that diet plays a role in both physical and mental disorders including anxiety, depression, behaviourial problems, major mental diseases such as schizophrenia, manic-depression and even delinquency and criminal behaviour. We only have to look at our present day lifestyle to see that it is very different to what nature intended for us. For example, most of us lead sedentary lifestyles with much less exercise and activity than we were intended to have. Our diets consist of foods which are highly processed and contain additives such as colourings, flavourings, preservatives, emulsifiers and so on. We have an excessive intake of sugar, salt, saturated fats and alcohol and of course these are known to contribute to degenerative diseases such as heart disease, diabetes, arthritis, cancer and psychiatric disorders.

Psychological and social factors, for example the loss of a loved one or chronic pain after a motor vehicle accident, may trigger off a stress reaction in which depression is the major element. These problems affect some people more than others. The psychological, physical and nutritional well-being of the person at the time of a major stress determines, to a significant degree, the outcome of the stress reaction. For example, if a person is reasonably well but suffers from mild headaches, mood swings, mild eczema or asthma at the time of a stressful event, their reaction to that event will probably be more severe than that of a person who is in very good health and symptom-free at the time of the stress.

Most of us are familiar with the normal mood swings which occur in everyday life. We know the sadness and dejection which can often arise from life's little disappointments and losses. These are of course normal to all of us and most of the time we cope with them reasonably well. Millions of people world-wide are now attempting to improve their physical health through diet, exercise, rest, meditation and other lifestyle changes. Many of these people have noted that by making some of these simple changes, they are more resistant to life's stresses and strains.

Those who have had physical or psychological illness in the past, discover a new lease of life with an increased ability to bounce back and block the devil of depression. They have found that the answer to many of their problems doesn't lie in complicated explanations of the psycho-dynamics and Freudian theories of depressive illness. Many have found that by simply removing certain foods from their diet or by adding exercise and a vitamin supplement, their mood swings and depressive illnesses become less severe and frequent over time.

CHAPTER THREE

The causes of tiredness

Introduction

WE ALL FEEL tired from time to time. Fatigue is a natural part of life and normally occurs at night at the end of a busy day. Fatigue and tiredness, like many bodily functions, is a cyclical phenomenon and it alternates with feeling alert and energetic. Fatigue only becomes a problem if it is severe and inappropriate, occurring at the wrong times of the day, and is persistent. The causes of tiredness, lethargy and fatigue are numerous and before a diagnosis of the chronic fatigue syndrome can be made other causes of this common symptom must be excluded.

Alfred's story

'I can't get through another day,' complained Alfred, a 56 year old business executive. For the past six months he had been complaining to his wife of increasing fatigue. She had encouraged Alfred to see a number of doctors for his condition but nothing physically could be found wrong in the way of heart or lung disease and blood tests showed Alfred was not anaemic.

Depression and stress from overwork in a very competitive engineering business was the conclusion of Alfred's local doctor. However, anti-depressants were of no help and a few changes to lifestyle, including more exercise and recreation did very little to improve Alfred's fatigue.

By this time Alfred had lost interest in everything. His hobby of photography had been abandoned. Life was miserable. He had been increasing his consumption of alcohol over the previous months in order to relax in the evenings. The drinks gave him a temporary feeling of well-being and more energy.

After intensive questioning, it seemed that the craving for alcohol was both physical and psychological. Although Alfred's blood glucose (blood sugar) levels had been found to be normal in previous tests, it was decided to perform a special glucose tolerance test to measure his body's ability to handle glucose (sugar).

It was discovered that Alfred's glucose tolerance test was abnormal and that he had a moderately severe form of adult onset diabetes. By simply changing his diet to one of complex carbohydrates, no alcohol or sugar and supplements of zinc, chromium and vitamin B-complex, dramatic changes occurred in his well-being, with far more energy available for work and exercise.

The causes of fatigue

1. The chronic fatigue syndrome
2. Medical causes of fatigue:
   Medically prescribed drugs, in particular tranquillisers, anti-depressants, blood pressure tablets, anti-epileptic medication, pain relieving medication, antihistamines, cortisone, some anti-inflammatory drugs
   Heart disease and early heart failure
   Diabetes

Lymphoma
Leukaemia
Liver disease
Kidney disease
Thyroid failure
Auto-immune disorders
Menopause
Arthritis (sometimes)

Chronic infections
Inflammatory disorders
Primary diseases of
   muscle
Myasthenia gravis
Multiple sclerosis
Adrenal failure

3. Psychological causes:
   Depression
   Anxiety
   Chronic stress reactions
   Schizophrenia

4. Nutritional causes of fatigue:
   Food allergies and food/chemical sensitivities
   Functional reactive hypoglycaemia (low blood sugar)
   Deficiencies of quality proteins, complex carbohydrates, essential fatty acids, vitamins, minerals or trace elements in the diet
   High sugar intake
   Alcohol
   Coffee
   Tea

5. Environmental causes of fatigue:
   Environmental pollutants including chemicals and heavy metals, such as mercury, lead, cadmium, arsenic.
   Pesticide and herbicide residues
   Electromagnetic radiation
   Jetlag
   The 'sick building' syndrome

6. Lifestyle factors causing fatigue:
   Over-training and over-exercising
   Sedentary lifestyle (unfitness)
   Irregular sleeping habits

Genetic resistance and susceptibility to disease

'Every winter I get two or three attacks of flu and I'm laid down for weeks. Antibiotics don't do me any good and I'm useless to anyone.'

These are the words often spoken by people frustrated with their high susceptibility to the common cold and influenza. Why do some people suffer endlessly with coughs, colds and bronchitis whilst others seemingly get away without a hint of illness. The genes we inherit from our parents play a very important role in the expression of the immune system and its ability to function. Of course, environmental factors including nutrition influence our state of health and the health of the immune system. It is highly likely that we all catch a similar number of colds and flus, but the responses of our system to the virus can vary greatly.

Host resistance to disease and its enhancement by natural means is the keystone to all good natural therapies. For example, in Indonesia children often contract severe respiratory or gastrointestinal infection and die as a consequence. The simple supplementation of a massive dose of vitamin A is sufficient to increase the resistance of the mucous membranes that lie in the nose, throat, lungs and gastrointestinal tract against the invasion of viruses and bacteria. Vitamin A is also known to play a role in the functioning of the immune cells. This is a classic example of manipulating one single variable to effect a dramatic result — the saving of young lives in Indonesia.

We are born with genes which we inherit from our parents and which inhabit the nucleus of every cell in our body. These genes are responsible for the expression of our physical make-up, such as the colour of our hair, eyes, the shape of our nose and whether we are male or female. The genes are also responsible for the functioning of the various cells, tissues and organs of the body. They determine the quality of protein we produce and they are responsible for the design and production of enzymes involved in the thousands of biochemical reactions occurring every second. It will therefore come as no surprise that the immune system's structure and functioning is determined to a large extent by the genes that are inherited. Our susceptibility to certain cancers, diabetes, heart disease and other health problems is to a large extent also determined by the genes that are inherited. Until recently, it was thought that the expression of these genes could not be affected by the environment, or manipulated by any outside forces. However, the science of genetic engineering has proven this precept incorrect. In the future we will see genes being inserted and removed from chromosomes in our cells to influence the course of disease.

Within the science of nutrition it is known that the enzymes and biochemical reactions determined by genetic expression can be influenced by the level of nutrients within the cell. Indirectly, this means that we can now alter to some degree the expression of genes we have inherited by nutritionally manipulating microenvironments of the cell. This is a very young science with great growth potential.

Inherited weakness in the immune system may not be severe enough to cause an immunological disease. However, immunological weakness can be improved by a change in diet and the use of therapeutic nutrition. Other important aspects of lifestyle play a role in immune expression as well. In the chapter on the mind we discuss how psychological and emotional stresses can profoundly suppress the immune system. The brain and the central nervous system produce some of the most potent and influential chemicals in the body. These chemicals may spread by nerves or in the bloodstream to different parts of the body to influence the functioning of many cells and organs. At times of physical or emotional stress, a disturbance in the balance of the various controlling chemicals from the central nervous system may play havoc with blood pressure, heart function, insulin output, glucose control and immune system functioning. These are only some of the bodily actions that may be affected by immune stress.

Should the immune system be chronically infected by a virus such as the Epstein-Barr virus, cytomegalovirus or coxsackie virus, the susceptibility of the nervous system, immune system and virtually every other cell in the body to stress is increased. This must be kept in mind during treatment programmes for people with the chronic fatigue syndrome because reactivation of these latent viruses is more frequent the higher the levels of stress. In fact, quite often the only symptom of sensitivity in the early stages

of an illness related to such a sensitivity is fatigue or tiredness.
 The organism that triggers fatigue in one victim may cause no more than a mild flu like illness or fever in other people, which is very strong evidence that the disease has a genetic and probably nutritional basis.

The causes of chronic fatigue syndrome

Primary

Heavy metal overload
Xenobiotic chemical overload or sensitivity.

Secondary

Nutritional deficiency and/or imbalance of nutrients
Chemical food sensitivity
Post viral syndrome — Epstein-Barr virus, cytomegalovirus, coxsackie B virus, glandular fever virus, influenza, chicken pox, German measles, mumps, measles, Human B-lymphotropic virus, Ross River virus
Bacterial infections
Candida albicans (thrush and other yeast infections)
Chronic stress weakening immune function
Functional reactive hypoglycaemia (low blood sugar)

Heavy metal overload resulting in fatigue-like symptoms

Most people living in western industrialised societies have all of these heavy metals in their systems, sometimes at significant levels: arsenic, excess copper, lead, mercury, aluminium, cadmium

Principal causes of the chronic fatigue syndrome, in order of importance

1. Heavy metal overload
2. Xenobiotic chemical overload
3. Borderline nutritional deficiencies
4. Food allergy and sensitivity

Heavy metals

The toxic heavy metals lead, mercury, arsenic, cadmium and aluminium are present in all of us to some degree. They are also present in patients with the chronic fatigue syndrome.

The two heavy metals that may play an important role in the suppression of the immune system and nervous system are lead and mercury. In 80% of the patients with the chronic fatigue syndrome significantly high levels of either lead or mercury are found in their tissues. Patients with the chronic fatigue syndrome have a total load of these heavy metals that is higher than the average. Blood tests for these toxic minerals are not as accurate as a hair or tissue analysis. In other words, the majority of patients with the chronic fatigue syndrome have significantly high levels of toxic metals in their system.

Lead poisoning has been known since ancient times and may have played a role in the fall of Rome when lead pewter was extensively used in eating and drinking utensils.

Lead poisoning is an insidious health problem and has gone unnoticed and undetected in many patients; its real importance has still not been realised in modern medicine. It has been described as the greatest nervous system poison and has become so widespread in our environment that its comparative effects are impossible to measure. Even the polar icecaps have shown an increase in lead levels of over 200 fold in the past 3,000 years. The lakes and oceans of the world contain up to twenty times more lead than they did prior to the industrial revolution.

People living in cities have 100 times more lead in their

bloodstream and up to 2,000 times more lead in their bones than before humans started using lead. The Roman Empire was the first civilised society to use lead in the lining of its wine casks, water containers and water reticulation systems. Observers noted that workers in lead smelters in ancient Rome suffered from unusual complaints, particularly relating to the nervous system. It is now believed by some historians and scientists that the actual decline of the Roman Empire may have been partially due to the result of a high intake of lead from water, foods and wine. It has certainly been documented that there was a decline of mental ability and a reduction in birth rates in ancient Rome.

Contamination of the environment with lead is ubiquitous and it is impossible to find an animal species that hasn't been exposed to it, so it is probably impossible to measure its real effect on humans. It may be that modern society is heading in the same downhill direction as ancient Rome . . .

Experiments in the laboratory show that even very low levels of lead can have an adverse effect on the nervous system. Once it has reached the nervous system, lead binds very strongly to nerve cells. Some scientists believe that there is no safe threshold for lead exposure and that once lead is present in the system its effects are irreversible.

Early signs of lead poisoning

1. Fatigue
2. Muscle pains
3. Impaired attention span and concentration
4. Poor short-term memory
5. Diminished language skills
6. Headaches
7. Poor co-ordination
8. Vertigo
9. Tremors
10. Indigestion and abdominal pains
11. Constipation
12. Pallor
13. Hyperactivity

It can be seen from the above that many of the symptoms of lead poisoning are common to those of the chronic fatigue syndrome — in particular fatigue, muscle aches and pains, poor concentration and attention span and the loss of short-term memory. Studies of children with lead poisoning demonstrate that they are more sensitive to lead and are more efficient at absorbing it into the body after ingestion. Studies of lead contamination in children show a direct relationship between the severity of symptoms including disturbances of brain function and the lead level in their blood.

Later signs of lead poisoning

1. Reduced intelligence quotient
2. Mental retardation
3. Signs of senility
4. Spontaneous abortion and still birth
5. ? Cancer
6. Kidney damage
7. Immune suppression
8. Premature death

Airborne lead is probably the major source of lead contamination in the environment, coming mainly from industry and the burning of leaded petrol in car exhaust fumes. Lead may also leech into domestic water supplied in older homes which often have lead pipes in their plumbing; this occurs more when the water is acidic. The weathering of lead containing paint, putty and other building materials in other homes can also contaminate household dust which can be swallowed or inhaled, particularly by young children. Children living in cities receive most of their lead from car exhaust fumes and from soil and dust that has been contaminated by chips of lead paint. Although the danger from lead in paints and car exhausts has been significantly reduced, the accumulation of lead over many years in the soil remains a significant problem. It has been estimated that the natural lead content of soil is approximately twenty parts per million. But in urban areas the soil near buildings in close proximity to busy highways may contain as much as ten thousand parts per million of lead.

It has been estimated that over 90% of the lead in the air in most modern cities is derived from automobile exhausts. Despite the change to lead free petrol, high octane fuels are still used and industry sources still remain a problem. Lead persists in the environment, in our bones and in our brains.

Lead can enter our food in a number of ways including lead soldered tin cans, improperly glazed dinnerware and even food supplements such as bonemeal and dolomite.

Occupational exposure is also possible, especially for workers in lead smelters and battery plants or exposed to hair dyes, although these are of course less common sources of contamination.

Sources of lead contamination

1. Leaded petrol (car exhaust fumes)
2. Food and water contaminated by atmospheric lead pollution
3. Pesticide sprays
4. Cooking utensils
5. Lead pipes
6. Lead paint in older homes (and lead in the dust)
7. Solders
8. Pigments
9. Batteries
10. Lead solder in tin cans

Many scientific studies have been conducted to show that dietary factors may protect to some degree against the toxic effects of lead. These include a high intake of plant food (fibre) and a number of vitamin and mineral supplements including vitamin C, B-complex vitamins, calcium, zinc, iron, chromium and copper; some of these nutrients actually decrease the absorption of lead.

Dietary nutrients can also reduce the accumulation of lead and prohibit the lead from binding to enzymes involved in normal metabolic processes. Animals treated with high doses of vitamin B1 have been shown to be protected against the harmful effects of lead. A controlled study of calves fed lead and vitamin B1 injections and another group of calves given lead only, indicated that vitamin B1 has a protective effect against lead poisoning. Signs of lead poisoning in this study were only apparent in untreated animals and these signs included weakness, disturbances in mobility, twisting of the spine and eventual blindness.

If high levels of lead are present in a hair analysis in a patient with the chronic fatigue syndrome, a therapeutic trial of high doses of vitamin B1 by injection, combined with the basic nutritional programme outlined in this book, is certainly worth considering. Vitamin B1 or thiamine is a very important co-factor in the metabolism of glucose to carbon dioxide, water and energy. In fact, the metabolism of carbohydrates is highly dependent upon an adequate supply of vitamin B1. It is possible, although not proven, that some of the enzymes requiring vitamin B1 for the metabolism of carbohydrates to energy, may in fact be blocked or poisoned by the presence of lead.

Another effective method of reducing the burden of lead is the use of EDTA chelation. Penicillamine, another chelating agent that can be used orally, may also be of benefit in some patients with the chronic fatigue syndrome who have not benefited significantly from other treatments. Penicillamine can be given orally under medical supervision. Regular blood tests are required for patients on penicillamine therapy to ensure that any toxic effects of the treatment are detected early. The toxic effects of penicillamine are significantly reduced when patients are treated concurrently with antioxidants and ascorbate.

Although it has not been definitely proven to be a major contributing factor to the chronic fatigue syndrome, the continued and increasing exposure to lead and its potential harmful effects on the immune system, nervous system and the endocrine glands must be taken seriously and, from the scientific evidence available, even comparatively low level exposures to lead prevailing in modern western societies interferes with metabolism.

Mercury toxicity and sensitivity

Hatmakers and dentists may seem worlds apart in their occupations but they have one thing in common. The hatmakers of the 19th century absorbed mercury through their skin and lungs from the felts used in hat making — mercuric nitrate was used in the felt-making process. 'Mad-Hatters disease', the 'Hatters Shakes' and other equally descriptive terms were used for the illnesses that hatmakers suffered. On the other hand, dentists work with amalgam dental fillings which contain a very high concentration of mercury. Exposure to mercury and mercury vapour, especially during the drilling and removal of old amalgams, is a potentially risky business for the dentist. Although the dental profession has yet to come to real terms with the possibilities of mercury toxicity both, to themselves and to their patients, some modern countries including Sweden, are banning the use of mercury amalgam.

Mercury is one of the most toxic substances known and its effects are definitely much less appreciated than they should be. The dental profession has an extremely high incidence of suicide worldwide — and when one examines the symptoms of mercury exposure one cannot help but ask the question 'Is mercury the cause or a contributing factor to dental suicide?'

Symptoms of mercury poisoning

1. Fatigue
2. Headache
3. Disturbances in short-term memory
4. Insomnia
5. Irritability
6. Depression
7. Personality deterioration
8. Numbness or tingling sensations of the fingers, toes and lips
9. Muscle weakness (this may progress to paralysis) — the cardinal symptom of CFS
10. Disturbances of co-ordination
11. Speech difficulties
12. Visual disturbances
13. Miscellaneous symptoms — fever, cough, chest pain, nausea, diarrhoea, abdominal cramps, skin rash
14. Toxic brain syndrome and insanity

Sir Isaac Newton, during his brilliant scientific career, apparently suffered a short period of insanity. It has been suggested that Newton suffered from mercury and lead poisoning as a consequence of working with mercury and its salts. A hair analysis of Newton's hair confirmed extremely high levels of mercury and lead.

The sources of mercury today are amalgams, food and air. Organic forms of mercury, such as methyl mercury, are more toxic than the metal itself and are present in our food supply. The history of widespread mercury poisoning goes back to 1953 when disabling neurological disorders began appearing in the Minamata district of Japan. Many people died and thousands became ill from mercury poisoning in this district as a consequence of a plastics factory dumping waste into the bay and polluting the local fish. The interesting thing in this story is that the local cats were the first to show signs of illness and behaviour disturbance before falling into a coma and dying. This illustrates how smaller living things can show signs of poisoning earlier than organisms higher up in the food chain.

We are now witnessing throughout the world a dramatic decline in the number of species surviving. It has been estimated that a species of animal or plant life is becoming extinct every five minutes. The warning signs are there and the present decline in some species of frogs should herald research into toxic heavy metal and herbicide and pesticide residues. Other reports of methyl mercury poisoning have occurred throughout the world not only due to fish poisoning but also to grains treated with organic mercurial fungicides.

It is the large fish, for example tuna and shark, that are the potential sources of mercury poisoning. The contamination of rivers, lakes and the sea by large chemical companies and paper manufacturers must be stopped. Shellfish and fish accumulate organic mercury — the larger the fish the greater the mercury contamination. At each step along the food chain the concentration of methyl mercury increases from plankton to algae to small marine creatures to small fish to larger fish and to the bigger fish. Organic mercury fungicides once used in agriculture may contaminate livestock and wild game also.

Mercury causes brain damage and other central nervous system disorders as well as birth defects. The toxic action of mercury is extensive. It binds to cell membranes, nuclear membranes, intracellular organelles and it inactivates enzymes essential for proper metabolism.

The issue of dental amalgams and their possible harmful effects remains controversial. However, significant anecdotal and scientific evidence in Australia, the United States and Great Britain supports the use of alternative dental materials in future. A patient suffering from the chronic fatigue syndrome who has tried diet and nutrient supplements with some benefit and who can be shown to have high levels of mercury or who is sensitive to mercury and its salts should seriously consider the total removal of dental amalgam. Thousands of lay people and many dental professionals have benefited from the removal of mercury from their teeth.

In 1988, scrap dental amalgam was declared a hazardous material by the United States Environmental Agency. Immediately a dentist removes an amalgam filling from the mouth and places it on a tray it once again becomes a hazardous and toxic waste material. The question should be asked — 'What is it about the mouth that makes the same substance apparently non-toxic.?' The answer is that this poison is not safe and statements that mercury amalgam is not harmful to the health is a gross misrepresentation.

It is important to know the facts behind mercury amalgam fillings. Mercury accounts for over 50% of the substances present in the silver amalgam. Worldwide research has shown that mercury vapour actually comes off a filling, particularly after stimulation through the chewing of foods, contact with hot or acidic foods, the brushing of teeth and by tooth grinding. Dentists and their professional associations have for decades advised that once mercury was placed with other ingredients in the dental fillings it was so tightly bound it could not escape. The other components of dental fillings include silver, tin, zinc and copper.

However, in the face of much research the dental profession has been forced to change that position and now admits that although mercury does come out of the filling, the amount according to them is insignificant. This is not so. Mercury is a known poison and that fact has been established for many years. In fact, mercury is such a strong, potent and penetrating poison that all living cells in the body are affected. It has not been shown to have any necessary biological function. According to some researchers, it is the single most toxic metal that has been investigated. Many authorities agree that mercury is even more toxic than lead, cadmium and arsenic. World regulatory agencies acknowledge that the minimum amount of mercury that will **not** cause damage is **unknown**. It thus remains an exercise in clear thinking in responding to the question, 'How can we be certain that the amount coming off dental fillings is insignificant?'.

Some of the world's foremost researchers on the toxicity of mercury and its salts conclude that the release of mercury from dental amalgams forms the predominant contribution to human exposure to inorganic mercury in the general population. In fact, the study of post mortem specimens actually shows a positive correlation between the number of occlusal surfaces of dental fillings and the levels of mercury in the kidneys and brain. Medical research has shown that mercury amalgams have an adverse effect on the number of T-cells in the immune system. It has also been demonstrated that the T-cells of the immune system return to normal after amalgams are carefully removed from the mouth. This is important in the chronic fatigue syndrome patients as they also have low T-lymphocyte levels. We must be careful here not to conclude that all T-lymphocyte reduction is due to mercury amalgams but we can conclude that it may be a significant factor. It is worth noting that amalgam restorations located on top of composite fillings, and not even in direct contact with the tooth, can result in a decrease in T-lymphocytes.

For those who believe that mercury amalgam is safe, let us examine another disease situation. The cerebrospinal fluid (CSF) - the fluid that surrounds the brain and spinal cord and bathes and supports it — has been shown to have eight times the level of mercury in patients suffering from multiple sclerosis when compared to healthy controls. This could be regarded as simply an interesting coincidence were it not for the fact that mercury is capable of producing symptoms that are indistinguishable from those of multiple sclerosis. Clinically large numbers of patients suffering from demyelinating encephalopathy (a multiple sclerosis-like syndrome), combined with a form of chronic fatigue, have responded extremely well to elimination diets, vitamin and mineral therapy and the removal of dental amalgams.

In the United States, the Environmental Protection Agency has declared that scrap dental amalgam is a hazardous waste material. Scrap amalgam is that portion of amalgam that remains after the dentist has placed a filling in the dental cavity. Dentists, according to the Materials Safety Data Sheet for mercury, are

advised to handle scrap amalgam extremely carefully. The following instructions are given to dentists:
1. Scrap amalgam must be stored in unbreakable, tightly sealed containers away from heat
2. A no-touch technique for handling amalgams should be used
3. Scrap amalgam must be stored under liquid, preferably glycerine or photographic fixant solution.

It can be seen that once an amalgam is removed from a tooth it again becomes a hazardous material and must be handled in the same way as scrap. If scrap amalgam has been carelessly disposed of the penalties are considerable. Again, we must ask the question, 'What is it about the mouth that makes mercury amalgam become non-toxic?' The logical response and the response by the non-professional lay public is that the danger persists.

The Alaskan Dental Association appropriated money for a paid advertisement entitled 'Straight Talk About Dental Amalgam' in April, 1989. They stated a number of facts, one being that 'The fillings in your teeth are safe. For more than a hundred years dentists have used, observed and tested amalgam filling material, and we have found them to be both safe and effective. No other material has been so thoroughly tested, nor found to be as cost effective as dental amalgams.' This statement by the Dental Association is misleading. Certainly, amalgam fillings have been tested for strength but not for their safety. The dental associations cannot produce definitive studies showing safety. Conversely, the research pointing to amalgam toxicity is exhaustive.

Interestingly, prior to the use of mercury amalgam fillings, it had been customary for many years to use lead fillings. These were also considered to be safe. In fact, the history of medicine is full of such anecdotes — toxic drugs are considered safe, radiation has been considered safe, the measurement of foot size by shoe fluoroscopy was considered safe and the routine use of pesticides and herbicides in increasing quantities are also considered safe. Only 25 years ago the medical associations supported the use of tobacco as an agent to help anxiety states.

The Alaskan Dental Association also stated, 'The dental profession has complete confidence in the safety of dental amalgam. The members of the dental team who work with amalgam everyday are as healthy as their peers and the general population. And most of us have — and would accept — amalgam fillings in our own mouths. Over one hundred million Americans have amalgam fillings.'

One must also examine the disturbances in neuropsychological functioning in over 90% of dentists tested. Neuropsychologists have shown areas of suboptimal function in many neurological tasks including attention span, the ability to concentrate, short-term memory, visual recall, disturbances in motor co-ordination, tremor and the perceptual accuracy in forming judgements. Certainly, a problem in any professional group. In the dentists tested, psychological problems were concentrated in the areas of irritability, impatience, tension, frustration and conflict. Notably absent was the measurement of calmness. It was observed that the longer a dentist practices, the less the ability he has to pass the entrance exams into dental school. Dentists should be informed of these studies showing the damage that is undermining their personalities and skills. It is also worth noting that amongst specialists dentists have the highest divorce and suicide rates. Of course, not all dentists will show signs of suffering because of individual differences but when 90% show signs of dysfunction, it is a problem for great concern.

One important point to be mentioned here is the slow, insidious onset of these symptoms. The change is so gradual that the damage may go unnoticed over a period of years. A comparison can be made between the rate of deterioration of eyesight and the rate of the appearance of mercury toxicity. A very slow, gradual loss of vision over many years is not detected on a day-to-day or week-to-week basis. A sudden loss of vision is dramatic. Therefore a very slow deterioration in eyesight or a very slow low-grade poisoning with amalgam go virtually unnoticed for a long time. The insidious nature of mercury toxicity fosters an uncertainty as to its true nature.

Another characteristic of mercury toxicity that has been substantiated by the Environmental Protection Agency is the association between women who are chronically exposed to mercury vapour, for example female dental personnel, and higher than normal spontaneous abortion rates, increased premature labour and greater perinatal mortality. Mercury has been shown to cross the placenta and assimilate itself into the fetus. Even the Californian Dental Association has established that significantly higher mercury levels are found in the placenta, membranes and the neonatal blood of women who are exposed to mercury while working in dental offices. In non-pregnant women there is a disturbance in the prevalence of the menstrual cycle and menstrual disorders. Spina bifida births (approximately 5%) occurred in one study population, the normal being less than .1%.

B-complex vitamins and folic acid have been shown to protect against the incidence of spina bifida and mercury is known to affect the function of folic acid in the body. The judicial use of folic acid, vitamin B12 and vitamin B-complex supplementation in women of childbearing years who have high levels of hair mercury should be an important consideration in preventative medicine.

According to the insurance statistics, dentists and dental personnel have one of the highest utilisation rates of medical insurance of any population. Mercury toxicity is generally not diagnosed as often as it should in the general population, or the dental profession. The reason for this is that early symptoms are generally non-specific and may vary greatly from one to another. This is exemplified in a case in which a dentist who suffered from numbness of the fingers was operated on surgically and treated for over fifteen years in several prestigious medical facilities before it was suspected that he may be suffering from mercury toxicity.

The diagnosis of mercury intoxication or mercury sensitivity is extremely difficult because of the insidious nature of the disorder and because most healthcare professionals are not familiar with proper diagnostic techniques. High levels of mercury may be found in the urine after acute exposure to the substance. However, normal levels of mercury in the urine are present in the majority of cases in which chronic low-grade exposure occurs. In fact, some experts believe that urinary mercury levels are characteristically low in chronic exposure, suggesting a hypersensitivity reaction. The levels of mercury in the urine are of limited value in the diagnosis of mercury poisoning. High levels can be found in people who are symptom free, and low levels may be detected in those with extensive symptoms of mercurial toxicity. This suggests that the failure to excrete mercury in the urine may be a factor in the development of poisoning. This exposes the fact that the relationship between urinary excretion of mercury and the absorbtion dose is not very well understood even by experts. The excretion of mercury via the kidney is dependent upon the health of the kidney. If the mercury has damaged the kidney function, excretion may be reduced. This results in the paradoxical situation in which only low levels of mercury appear in the urine in the mercury toxic or sensitive individual. Some workers in the field have found that the longer a worker was on a job in which mercury exposure was high the less mercury they excreted in their urine.

Blood tests are also not very helpful in the diagnosis of mercury poisoning since the metal remains in the blood for a few minutes only and quickly deposits itself in the brain, adrenals, thyroid glands, pituitary gland and kidneys. As one doctor specialising in this field in the United States has commented, 'There are not enough words to describe the dentists and dental assistants I have seen whose lives have been devastated by the effects of chronic mercury exposure. It is truly heartbreaking - and preventable!'.

The fact that over one hundred million people have mercury fillings in their mouths does not mean that it is necessarily safe and right. The majority is not always right.

Facts on dental amalgam

1. Amalgam consists of 50% mercury
2. Approximately 80% of the world's dental caries are filled with amalgam
3. Mercury vapours are released from amalgam restoration
4. Twelve or more amalgams produce 29 micrograms of mercury per day
5. One to four amalgams produce 9 micrograms of mercury per day
6. The above levels of mercury exceed accepted standard of exposure
7. 80% of the mercury can be absorbed through the lungs
8. Un-ionized mercury vapour can pass directly to the brain

9. Mercury is an accumulative metal in tissues
10. The brain content of mercury is related to the number of amalgam fillings
11 Many symptoms improve following amalgam removal
12. Students with amalgams have 45% more health symptoms than students without them
13. Chronic low doses of mercury can be very harmful to health

Another fact stated by the Alaskan Dental Association was 'Any dentist who encourages you to remove amalgam fillings in order to remove toxic substances from the body is guilty of a breach of ethics. In addition to the ADA, the United States Public Health Services, the National Institute of Dental Research and the Consumers Union have all investigated the allegations about amalgam — and have found them to be useless.'

Remember, the ADA formerly maintained that mercury did not come out of the filling. This has been shown to be totally incorrect. Furthermore, a dentist who is subject to a breach of dental ethics for suggesting that mercury is toxic, may actually remove the filling for cosmetic reasons without the threat of censure or removal of his licence. Clearly, there is a distortion of judgement if it is held to be unethical to remove a documented biological poison from the mouth whilst it is ethical to actually place this substance there in the first place.

The various dental authorities worldwide have held 'There is no scientifically documented evidence of a cure or improvement of a specific disease due to the removal of mercury amalgam restoration from non allergenic patients.' This is probably true to a point because mercury toxicity and sensitivity is not a specific disease. Nevertheless, thousands of cases treated by doctors of nutritional and environmental medicine in England, Europe, the United States, Canada and Australia have been documented testifying to improvements in the chronic fatigue syndrome, hormonal disturbances, neurological diseases, anxiety and depression, epileptiform conditions, visual problems, headaches, irritability, ideas of suicide, phobias, muscle aches and pains, joint pains, irritable bowel syndrome, cardiac abnormalities, skin rashes, acne-like disorders after the removal of amalgams.

The truth is that nobody fully appreciates the ramifications of dental amalgam on human health.

Decisions about amalgam fillings, like all decisions made about dental health, should be able to be made in the dentist's surgery within the bounds of the doctor-patient relationship. However, this is somewhat difficult. Patient enquiries about what material is being placed in their mouth and its safety are often left with the response, 'There is no scientific evidence that it causes disease.'

Improvements in non-mercury fillings with new composite material have occurred over the last few years. There is no reason now why a dentist should use mercury amalgam in preference to a composite resin. The composites may not have the durability of mercury amalgam but they are far safer.

The forward thinking Swedish Government Health Board has declared amalgam toxic and unsuitable as a dental filling material. Public hearings in Sweden towards the end of 1988 reinforced and upheld that ruling. Many dentists now have seriously questioned the status quo regarding the safety of mercury amalgams.

The removal of old fillings requires special training and techniques including the use of rubber dams and special exhaust and draining equipment to ensure the minimal exposure to mercury vapours to both the patient and the dentist. Tests on possible allergy reactions to various dental materials can be performed prior to the replacement of old amalgam with new filling materials. This can reduce the necessity for sometimes a second or third removal of incompatible restoration material.

Symptoms in the mouth suggestive of amalgam incompatibility

1. A metallic taste
2. A salty taste
3. Tingling or burning of the tongue or gums
4. Sensitivity of the pulp (the soft part in the centre of the tooth containing blood vessels and nerves)
5. Excessive secretion of saliva
6. Recurrent mouth ulcers
7. Neuralgia in or around the mouth
8. Loss of sense of taste or smell

What can be done to protect against mercury toxicity and sensitivity? Firstly, the presence of mercury toxicity or a hypersensitivity state must be assessed and can be performed by special tests including a full hair analysis, immunological tests, blood tests, a urine measurement after EDTA chelation therapy and special electronic tests for hypersensitivity states. Certain dietary fibres including alginates and pectin may offer some help against inorganic mercury poisoning but they have minimal influence on methyl mercury. Scientific studies have shown that the trace element selenium binds to tissue sites and blocks the effect of both organic and inorganic mercury poisoning and protects against most of mercury's toxic effects. The use of vitamin C and zinc helps with some of the symptoms of mercury sensitivity as does high potency B-complex vitamins. Intravenous ascorbate may also help as a weak chelating agent and if this is unsatisfactory then the use of EDTA or dimercaprol (BAL) are suitable drug alternatives. Penicillamine is another chelating agent of use in acute cases of mercury poisoning.

To achieve a therapeutic response using selenium (as sodium selenite) as a mineral antagonist to methyl mercury high doses of selenium are necessary. Doses in the range of 1,000 to 2,000 micrograms of elemental selenium per day may be necessary for four to eight weeks initially to achieve a response. These extremely high levels of selenium intake must eventually be reduced to approximately 200 to 400 micrograms of selenium per day. During this time careful blood tests and monitoring of selenium levels are essential to avoid toxic effects of the selenium in the patient.

The bottom line in the chronic fatigue syndrome patient is how well the patient feels at the end of the day. If all the simple measures outlined in this book have been faithfully carried out and problems are persistent it is worth seriously considering the use of total amalgam clearance using appropriate dams and high volume extraction water spray plus appropriate chelation therapy. The patient has very little to lose and much to gain.

An important question remains and that is 'What are the health effects that occur after the removal of dental amalgam?'.

Case history

> Janice Wilson had been under the care of a psychiatrist for three years because of her suicidal tendencies, trying to figure

out what had happened in her childhood that made her so angry with herself and the world. Janice had been seen by many doctors and specialists including neurologists for her poor co-ordination, dizzy spells, confusion and generalised pains in the back and spinal regions. She had suffered from blackouts, nausea and severe migraines, more pronounced on the days in the middle of her menstrual cycle. Recently, severe tinnitus or ringing in the ears had developed and made her depression even more intolerable.

At the suggestion of a friend, Janice visited a doctor specialising in nutritional and environmental medicine and it was discovered that abnormal electrical currents occurred between a number of amalgams in her teeth. It was also demonstrated that she had a sensitivity to organic mercury and therefore it was decided to carefully remove all amalgam fillings.

Some three months after the removal, most of her chronic symptoms had improved and many had disappeared completely. The depression and suicidal thoughts cleared up and Janice was able to return to a happier and more productive lifestyle.

Case history

The following case history is a report taken from the medical literature to show just how dramatic mercury amalgam toxicity can be and how equally dramatic the relief of symptoms can be after its removal.

A 17 year old girl had dropped out of school due to health problems. More than 45 healthcare professionals had been involved in this case and none could help her. She suffered from excruciating attacks of pain in the chest that lasted for up to three hours at a time, accompanied by a feeling of impending doom. It was documented that these severe chest pains commenced shortly after dental amalgam fillings had been placed in her mouth six months earlier. Almost immediately following the amalgam filling she became introverted, psychiatrically disturbed and suffered from hallucinations, back and chest pains, shortness of breath, suicidal ideas and she developed an abnormal red coloured rash from the waist upwards. Within one week after the amalgam was removed, all of her symptoms had subsided.

Continuing the health effects after the removal of amalgam

One study on 86 subjects who had their amalgams removed revealed that a total of 70% of symptoms were either eliminated completely or greatly improved. These included symptoms referrable to the skin, cardiovascular system, nervous system, digestion, blood pathology tests, hormonal symptoms, psychological symptoms, allergies and a variety of other diseases. It was found that within an average of 10 months after amalgam removal nearly 70% of symptoms were either improved or eliminated. Following the removal of amalgam approximately 80% of subjects claimed that they felt better and over 90% said that they would repeat the procedure. Nearly 60% of patients claimed an increase in happiness and peace of mind and the overall well-being of most subjects improved considerably after amalgam removal.

These results greatly exceed the benefits expected if only the placebo response was operating, indicating that the effects of the removal are significant.

How does mercury poison?

There a number of theories about how mercury causes toxicity or sensitivity symptoms. Pure inorganic mercury may be directly toxic to the bodies tissues. Organic salts, for example methyl mercury, may cause sensitivity symptoms and allergies in the immune system.

Proteins contain special molecules called sulfhydryl groups which are essential for their proper function. Mercury is highly reactive and can combine with these sulfhydryl groups therefore inactivating them and their proteins. If the protein is a structural protein in a cell membrane, then the structure of that organ is affected. If the mercury attaches to a sulfhydryl group on a protein enzyme then the activity of the enzyme is reduced. Therefore, in this way mercury can affect structural tissue proteins, hormones, enzymes and transmitters within the nervous and immune system. Mercury only has to react with a very small number of key reactive centres containing sulfhydryl groups to cause widespread damage and toxicity. Hence, mercury can destroy cell membranes, nuclear membranes, cytoplasmic organelles, mitochondria, chromosomes, in fact nearly every important part of a living cell. Mercury may stimulate the formation of highly reactive free radicals which are extremely damaging to the macromolecules in the cell. They cause unnecessary oxidation reactions resulting in the rancidification of the bodies fats and oils (lipids).

Mercury has also been shown to interfere with the immune system and over 60% of the allergy symptoms, including fatigue, are either improved or eliminated completely after amalgam removal.

Allergic skin reactions are more frequent if amalgams have been left in the mouth for more than five years.

Mercury also plays a role in many autoimmune diseases. Autoimmune diseases are those diseases in which the immune system produces antibodies that attack tissues and organs to cause degeneration. For example, autoantibodies to a person's thyroid gland can cause the thyroid gland to fail. Antibodies to the pancreas have been demonstrated in patients with diabetes. It is thought that even multiple sclerosis may be an auto-immune disease secondary to a disturbance of the immune system caused by a number of possible factors in combination including a viral infection, mercury toxicity, vitamin or mineral deficiencies and excessive free radicals. Multiple sclerosis is a disease in which the nerves of the brain and spinal chord lose their protective myelin coat. Mercury is known to cause this loss of myelin also.

The T-lymphocytes in the blood are special white blood cells that play an important role in the immune system. Following the placement of mercury amalgam these T-lymphocytes often decrease in number. After removal of the amalgam, the T-lymphocytes return to normal. These T-lymphocytes are also found to be depressed in numbers in patients with the chronic fatigue syndrome. Some patients with the chronic fatigue syndrome who have had their mercury amalgam removed and who have improved in health have also shown an increase in their

T-lymphocytes. The T-lymphocytes are important in that they protect against viruses and yeasts. Again, we see in the chronic fatigue syndrome more viral infections and certainly more problems with yeasts especially the yeast that causes thrush, known as candida albicans. Thus it becomes apparent that many factors play a role in the destruction of health in the patient with the chronic fatigue syndrome.

Electric currents in the mouth

Small electric currents can be generated between different metals placed in the fillings of the mouth. Some healthcare workers believe that these electrical currents can have widespread effects on the mouth, the nerves of the oral cavity and the central nervous system. Indirectly, these influences may cause disturbances elsewhere in the body.

Small electromagnetic fields may affect mental and physical health by disrupting the electromagnetic fields of individual cells. Some dentists now advise patients to have these electromagnetic fields evaluated by using electro probes and current metres. This is a highly specialised form of diagnosis and must be left to experienced operators. It may be that these small electromagnetic fields are responsible for the stress-like symptoms in the nervous system including anxiety, depression, irritability, anger and phobias. All of these symptoms are associated with mercury poisoning.

One final comment about the removal of amalgams. Some symptoms may temporarily become worse in the immediate period following removal. This is probably due to minute quantities of mercury leeching into the bloodstream and nervous system. Some opponents to the removal of mercury amalgams argue that the improved health benefits and reduction of symptoms is due to the placebo affect. If this were the case, why do some symptoms become much worse before they get better after amalgam removal? When this question is put to the supporters of amalgam there is no satisfactory answer. The fact remains that tens of thousands of people with sometimes extremely severe health problems have gained dramatic benefit from the removal of mercury from their mouths.

Sweden's banning of mercury amalgam for future use in dentistry must surely delight those who see the careless indiscriminate use of heavy metals and other chemicals as a threat to the health of the planet.

CHAPTER FOUR

Viruses, bacteria and candida

The Epstein-Barr virus (EBV)

A viral cause has been the major focus for research into the chronic fatigue syndrome. However, as previously mentioned, a variety of other predisposing factors may co-exist which permit, allow or promote the proliferation of the virus and/or its effects. The virus implicated in a large majority of patients with the chronic fatigue syndrome is the Epstein-Barr virus (EBV). This a large DNA-Virus which belongs to the family of herpes viruses. It is probably responsible for most cases of glandular fever also known as infectious mononucleosis, and it has been associated with a cancer of the lymph glands called Burkitt's lymphoma and cancer of the nasal cavity. Another virus of the same family called cytomegalovirus (CMV) has been implicated in glandular fever type diseases as well. Many other viruses probably have the potential to cause chronic fatigue syndrome but most patients with the severest symptoms have either EB virus or CMV.

Susceptible youth

The majority of people in the western world are exposed to the Epstein-Barr virus before the age of thirty. However, in underdeveloped countries, exposure of the population occurs before adolescence and it generally occurs during early childhood. This leads to a subclinical infection which is similar to a mild flu-like illness.

As in the western world, if the infection occurs during adolescence or young adulthood, a more prolonged and severe illness follows. Generally this is the classical picture of acute glandular fever with severe weakness, debility, fever, sweats, enlargement of lymph glands in the neck, armpits and groin and enlargement of the liver and sometimes also the spleen. It is during this acute stage of a flu-like or viral illness, especially of the glandular fever type, in which massive doses of intravenous vitamin C are most effective in aborting the illness. From clinical experience gained from thousands of patients, acute viral illnesses respond dramatically to intravenous ascorbate treatment.

A lifetime companion

Whether the infection occurs during childhood, or in adolescence and adulthood, the virus appears to persist for life. For most of us who are in general good health and adequately nourished, this chronic carrier state is of little consequence. The reactivation of the virus within the immune system and its associated organs may occur in some people. This results in either acute bouts of viral infection and/or a chronic low grade illness, including severe fatigue that is often extremely debilitating. Other factors including genetics, geographical distribution, poor diet and the co-existence of other infections seem to play a role in the reactivation of this virus. In fact the propensity to develop Burkitt's lymphoma is extremely high in the malarial areas of Africa. The cancer of the nasal cavity mainly effects the Eskimos, Chinese and North Africans from specific regions. The persistence of the Epstein-Barr virus in chronically infected people probably reflects a weakness of the immune system. This weakness may come about as a consequence of a genetic susceptibility, poor nutrition, the co-existence of other viral, bacterial or fungal infections, an overload of toxic pollutants and perhaps even the production of immune chemicals by the individual's body cells themselves. These 'immune chemicals' may have a virus-activating effect.

It is known that chemicals produced by the nervous system and the adrenal glands in a person under stress, can be converted in the body to highly reactive free radicals. These free-radicals are very damaging to the cells of the body and attack macromolecules such as proteins, DNA, RNA and the unsaturated lipids present in every cell and tissue of the human body. Therefore, an effective management strategy for a patient with CFS requires an approach which will address all these possible causative or aggravating factors. Their recovery is dependent upon an effective and specific immune response by so-called cytotoxic T-cells, helper cells and suppressor cells of the immune system.

The EB virus appears to persist in the B cells which are the major antibody producing cells of the immune system. Therefore the effective inhibition of the virus requires a cell-mediated response in order to inhibit the reproduction of the EB virus plus the destruction of virally infected cells. This is an extremely complex picture to understand and it is complicated even further by the fact that the antibody producing cells which produce antibodies to eliminate virus infections are themselves infected by the virus. There are special cells of the immune system called killer cells (NK cells) and they are capable of targeting and destroying other virally infected cells.

Another important cell-line of the immune system is the Suppressor Cell line. These cells, known as T8 cells, secrete chemical substances which have the ability to switch off overactive or abnormal conditions of the immune system. They may also inhibit the function of the virally infected B cells.

Rosetta's candida

> At 35, Rosetta believed she had accomplished much. 'I have my own home, a child, a good job, my own car, I own real estate and I've done it all on my own,' she explained.
>
> But now the crunch had come. Rosetta regularly ate in restaurants with business associates and friends and she also liked a glass or two of wine. Her favourite foods were

red meats, roasted potatoes and, to finish off the meal, varieties of cake. Over the previous few winters Rosetta had suffered from a number of viral infections and was recently laid up in bed for three weeks with swollen glands and a fever. Following this, severe bouts of fatigue persisted to the point where working was impossible.

It was discovered that Rosetta had suffered from vaginal thrush (candida) on and off for most of her adult life and when it was active her health was affected. Combined with the fatigue, this reactivated vaginal thrush was sufficient to throw Rosetta almost into a panic.

Having been placed on a low refined carbohydrate diet free of added yeast and complete elimination of alcohol, she discovered to her amazement that not only did the candida disappear but her fatigue remarkably improved.

The only problem that remained was the dramatic change to her lifestyle and social life. Rosetta found it hard to face meals without her wine and sweets and she would punish herself from time to time by breaking her diet and bingeing. She realised that it sometimes took a week or two to recover from a binge and after six months of coaxing and manipulation and juggling, she finally decided to stick to her diet for twelve months to allow herself enough time for a full recovery.

Eventually Rosetta found that she could take small quantities of sugar and have a glass of alcohol provided she kept to her diet fairly strictly most of the time.

Promotion of virus reproduction

All these functions of the immune system are totally dependent on a healthy internal environment plus an optimum supply of essential nutrients. A number of environmental factors have been discovered which actually promote the Epstein-Barr Virus infection, including synthetic chemicals. Tung Oil is a drying oil obtained from the seeds of the tree Aleurites. This oil is a valuable ingredient in varnishes and is used in many wood-working products, paints, construction materials and even in the manufacture of clothing. The Tung Oil not only promotes the EB virus infection by activating it but it is a known immunosuppressive agent also. The actual ingredients in the Tung Oil appear to be a number of phorbol esters. Similar compounds are found both naturally and in synthetics, and therefore the generalisation is made that exposure to all substances must remain guarded in the individual with chronic fatigue syndrome and Epstein-Barr virus infections.

Herbal compounds are generally regarded as being safe and in many cases effective in the management of many illnesses, symptoms and diseases. However, some herbs which have been used both by western and chinese healers, have actually been shown to activate viruses. These include angelica, euphorbia, clematis intricata and datura stramonium (Jimson Weed) and possibly large doses of other herbal remedies known to have an anti-inflammatory effect including feverfew, devil's claw and echinacea.

Our genes influence virus infections

It is highly probable that genetics play a role in the susceptibility of the individual to chronic viral infections such as EBV and CMV. Research data is consistent with this concept, but it is unclear as to the exact degree of that contribution. It is known that in some people with inherited severe immune deficiency states that there is evidence of a chronic EBV infection in their system. Two such rare diseases are ataxia-telangiectasia and the Wiskott-Aldrich syndrome.

More on the Epstein-Barr Virus and cytomeglovirus

The Epstein-Barr virus is a member of the herpes group of viruses that include herpes simplex — the cause of cold sores and genital herpes or ulcers of the membranes of the penis and vagina. The herpes group of viruses also contain the chicken pox virus, cytomeglovirus and the virus which is responsible for shingles (herpes zoster). All of these viruses have the ability to establish a chronic or lifelong infection in the patient's body. The virus usually remains inside the cells of the immune system and sometimes the cells of the liver, spleen and lymph glands of the body. Of course, without an efficiently functioning immune system this quiescent and persistent inhabitation of the host cells would result in further infection and illness.

Should the immune system of the host be compromised in any way, this so-called 'latent infection' may become activated. When this happens, the immune system's ability to suppress virus replication becomes less effective and virus particles therefore multiply and spread within the host. This phenomenon occurs readily in herpes infections. Many people who suffer from cold sores know that at times of extra emotional or physical stress, exposure to sunlight, illness or even after excessive alcohol consumption, an attack of the cold sores is more likely to occur. In AIDS patients whose immune systems are infected with the HIV virus the same thing happens. Under any stress, the AIDS virus seems to take advantage and multiply extremely rapidly, resulting in widespread damage to the patient's immune system, nervous system and gastrointestinal tract. Glandular fever is another good example. Under stress, teenagers and young adults may suffer from relapsing illness from severe and persistent symptoms including fatigue, sweaty fevers and enlargement of lymph glands in the neck, armpits and groin.

The spread of the virus generally occurs via saliva and during close contact as in, for example, kissing. This is why the disease glandular fever or infectious mononucleosis is sometimes referred to as the kissing disease. The virus in the saliva can be persistent and it may last for twelve months after the glandular fever-like illness has disappeared. In a few individuals, the virus may persist even longer and perhaps indefinitely.

Glandular fever (infectious mononucleosis)

This is probably one of the most common causes of the chronic fatigue syndrome, especially in young adults. In fact, this most debilitating viral infection in young adults has resulted not only in chronic illness, but severe psychiatric and social disturbances also. The most effective method of controlling this illness is in the early stages. At the first sign of a glandular fever-like illness, the rapid administration of megadose vitamin C by mouth and, if necessary, by injection intravenously, is dramatic in not only relieving the symptoms but reducing the size of the glands and liver, which are often quite enlarged. Vitamin C, as discussed elsewhere, is not only a potent viral inhibitor but also a very important immune-system stimulator and antioxidant. Thus it not only inhibits virus replication in the patient but it improves both cellular and humeral immunity while simultaneously detoxifying the system from the excess of any chemicals, drugs or antibiotics that may have been prescribed.

The immune system chemicals include interferons and interleukins and their breakdown products which may act as free-radicals. These may in themselves be responsible for symptoms and immune dysfunction. The immediate administration of intravenous vitamin C is often dramatic. Combined with an intramuscular injection of high potency B-complex, folic acid and 1000mcg of vitamin B12, patients who are almost moribund from the illness may turn around within two hours and become almost symptom free. However, the administration of intravenous and intramuscular vitamins must continue for a week to ten days to ensure maintenance of this state of well-being.

A lesson to be learned here is that the longer the delay between onset of a patient's symptoms and the administration of intramuscular and intravenous vitamins, the longer it takes to achieve an improvement in their condition. Of course, other immune supporting nutrients must be administered orally as soon as possible after the diagnosis of the disease is made.

Glandular fever most commonly occurs in young adults and students between the ages of 15 and 23 years. If severe, it may have a profound effect on the individual's immediate and future life. The period between the time of initial infection and the onset of symptoms, which is known as the incubation period, may be as long as two to three months. Therefore, it is often difficult to go back in the history of the illness and determine the exact source or time of infection.

An indication that a glandular fever-like illness has occurred he mild symptoms which become apparent at the initial stages of the illness. These include headache, weakness, fatigue, muscle pains and sore throat with a mild flu-like illness. This may occur two to six weeks prior to the actual onset of the severe debilitating glandular fever. It is then that the severe fever, weakness, fatigue, extreme sore throat and enlargement of the glands in the front and back of the neck occur. Enlargement of the liver, and sometimes the spleen, may occur with a flat red rash on the trunk. This rash is brought on by drugs such as ampicillin. The hallmarks of glandular fever are the severe pharyngitis or sore throat and the generalised enlargement of the lymph glands in the neck, armpits, elbow regions and groin. Although liver enlargement does occur, it is unusual. However, on testing liver function it is nearly always abnormal.

In the blood tests we find an increase in the number of all types of white cells, plus an increase in abnormal lymphocytes. A positive test for glandular fever doesn't occur until about three weeks after the onset of the symptoms. Therefore the diagnosis must be made on the clinical picture alone, at least in the early stages. The use of antibiotics and other drugs in patients with acute glandular fever and liver dysfunction is unwarranted and may even aggravate the situation. With the liver malfunctioning, detoxification of xeniobiotic chemicals is comprised and the possibility of making a patient sensitive to foods and chemicals by prescribing antibiotics and drugs is high. The only treatment, as mentioned before, is the use of intravenous vitamin C, intramuscular high potency B-complex with B12 and folic acid and oral supplementation including B-complex, zinc and appropriate supportive herbal and homeopathic remedies. This natural medicine approach is advocated to improve the immediate situation and reduce the possibility of complications such as chronic Epstein-Barr virus infection, Non-A Non-B hepatitis, liver damage, infections of the nervous system and heart and the possibility of developing lymphoma.

Chronic Epstein-Barr virus infection is a disease now known to be associated with the persistent symptoms of chronic fatigue syndrome. In fact, the persistence of elevated antibodies towards various viral antigens in individuals suffering from the chronic fatigue syndrome is indirect evidence that this virus at least plays a part in the production of the disease.

EB virus associated diseases

Re-occurring or chronic Epstein-Barr virus infections have been found in a number of disease states. The diseases in which chronic EBV is found are generally diseases in which the immune system is suppressed, compromised or stressed in such a way that it functions subnormally. These diseases include of course AIDS and AIDS-related complexes, leukaemia, some cancers, lymphoma and Hodgkin's disease. It may also occur in such disorders as SLE (systemic lupus erythematosis), rheumatoid arthritis, ankylosing spondylitis, multiple sclerosis and in renal transplant patients who have received immunosuppressive drugs.

Other drugs which may suppress immune function and permit the persistence of EB virus infection include cortisone therapy and chemotherapeutic drugs used in suppressing cancer growth. In raising the question about the Epstein-Barr virus's involvement in these disorders, two possible propositions emerge. Firstly, is the presence of the Epstein-Barr virus and its reactivation the result of a damaged or malfunctioning weakened immune system or, secondly, is the Epstein-Barr virus in itself the major factor creating the damaged immune state? It is extremely difficult to answer this vexing question and for the time being it must be regarded as a chicken and egg situation. The most likely scenario is that a weakened or stressed immune system is attacked by one or more of these viruses and, unable to completely resolve the infection, it cannot eradicate the virus from the immune cells. As a consequence, the virus becomes firmly established within the immune cells and persists, eventually damaging their fine metabolic machinery. This results in a continual, gradual weakening of the entire immune system. Along comes another stress such as some physical trauma, a viral infection or an overload of chemical pollution and the weakened immune system is further compromised, unable to contain the chronic viral infection. EB virus then commences to replicate and do further damage. This process is cyclical and continues until such a point is reached when the immune system fails completely and an end stage auto-immune disease, inflammatory disorder or cancer occurs.

Although hypothetical, this proposition is the most likely and is an extremely good model to work from clinically. It offers the health practitioner the opportunity to strengthen the immune system through appropriate lifestyle changes and thus minimise the likelihood of the downward spiral to disease.

Another extremely interesting facet of the chronic EB virus infection is the association with other viruses. It has been found, for example, that of individuals who suffer from the chronic fatigue syndrome and who have Epstein-Barr virus antibodies, those with the most severe illness have the highest levels of antibodies to EB virus. This group with severest fatigue and highest antibodies also have high levels of antibodies to the herpes viruses, measles and cytomegalovirus (CMV). Here again, one suspects weakening of the immune system by one virus resulting in easier infection by a number of other viruses which further weaken the immune system's resistance. Some scientists now suggest, with strong evidence to support their case, that vaccination may itself weaken the immune system or make it susceptible in some way to the carrier virus state.

Characteristics of chronic viral infections

1. Infections may last for life
2. May weaken the immune system
3. Stress may reactivate the virus
4. Many other viral infections may develop
5. Chronic weakening of immune function may result in autoimmune disease, lymphoma, leukaemia or cancer
6. Susceptibility to food and chemical sensitivity is greater because of immune-dysfunction

Making the diagnosis

When, as is usually the case, physical examination reveals no obvious abnormality and routine pathology tests, blood tests, X-rays etc. are negative, it is difficult for the doctor or practitioner to accept CFS as a proper medical diagnosis. Doctors tend to believe their tests in the establishment of a diagnosis often in preference to what they have been told in the history-taking exercise.

To emphasize again, the major symptom of CFS is severe muscle fatigue following minimal or minor muscular activity, from which it may take hours or even days to recover. This fatigue may prevent the patient from even getting out of bed or, if they do, sitting at a table or watching television may itself become a tiring exercise. In fact, watching television may aggravate the problem because of electromagnetic pollution. Even reading the paper or a book may result in fatigue to the arms, eyes and neck muscles. In other words, a life without energy.

Other symptoms which appear in time and should be regarded as complicating the disorder include headaches, muscle aches and pains, joint aches and pains, muscle twitching, irritability, nausea, painful glands, loss of short-term memory, apathy, anxiety, depression, emotional instability, a ringing in the ears and abnormal sensations in the fingers or toes.

For the diagnosis of CFS to be accepted by the medical profession, the fatigue must have persisted for at least six months or longer. It is indeed unfortunate that a patient must wait an extra two or three months after suffering from fatigue for three or four months before their condition is taken seriously enough to make a diagnosis. As will be explained later, the earlier that treatment is commenced after fatigue sets in, the better is the individual's prognosis. Also, patients respond more rapidly to dietary and lifestyle changes the earlier that they are implemented.

It is interesting to note in this group of individuals with CFS that the symptoms of neurosis and depression are generally not as severe as the psychological symptoms are in the typical psychiatric patient suffering from severe depression or anxiety.

Controlled scientific studies have revealed that a significant number of patients with the chronic fatigue syndrome sometimes have a dramatic reduction in the number of white blood cells and special immune cells called lymphocytes in their blood. Although there is no definite diagnostic test for CFS, the criteria for its diagnosis have been established.

Medically accepted diagnostic criteria for CFS

1. A chronic, relapsing, severe muscular fatigue which is exacerbated by minimal exertion and which causes a significant disruption of the usual daily activities. This fatigue must have been present for six months or longer.
2. A disturbance in function of the nervous system with psychiatric symptoms including impairment of concentration and reduction in short-term memory revealed by difficulties in completing mental tasks which had normally been accomplished with ease.
3. An abnormal cell-mediated immune response evidenced by a reduction in the numbers of helper and suppressor lymphocytes (T4 and T8 cells of the immune system) and/or a lack of response in delayed type sensitivity skin tests (tests similar to the skin tests for tuberculosis).

It has been observed under the very powerful electron microscope that the red blood cells of patients suffering from chronic fatigue syndrome are unstable and become distorted. This distortion is worse at times when patients are suffering from severe fatigue and the cells may even return to normal when the patients are feeling reasonably well. This intermittent disturbance to the red blood cells may be a manifestation of damage to the very sensitive red blood cell membrane which surrounds the cell and maintains its normal saucer shape. It has been postulated, and is highly probable, that damage to the red blood cell membrane is caused by free-radicals and other oxidising chemicals attacking the membranes. Their increased susceptibility may be due to genetic and nutritional factors and a lack of sufficient antioxidants in the membranes themselves. The normal red blood cell is responsible for the delivery of oxygen to the tissues and removal of carbon dioxide wastes and organic acids from the bodies tissues. If there is a disturbance in the function of the red blood cell and its activity, the possibility of reduced oxygen transport by red blood cells and therefore oxygen starvation to the tissues is likely. This may explain why some of the oxygenation techniques used in treating the chronic fatigue syndrome have been effective in hundreds and perhaps thousands of patients worldwide. These oxygenation techniques are discussed elsewhere.

Before the definitive diagnosis of CFS is made, the doctor needs to exclude all other organic diseases. A full blood examination and haemoglobin level is necessary to eliminate blood disorders and anaemia and thyroid function tests, liver function tests and kidney function tests should also be performed.

It is also essential to rule out the unlikely possibility of a malignancy, cancer or leukaemia and any specific neurological disease such as multiple sclerosis. A blood glucose and extended glucose test may be necessary if diabetes or functional reactive hypoglycaemia are suspected.

The fatigue chemicals

Interferon is a chemical produced by the white cells called lymphocytes in the blood, in response to infection by a virus. Interferon may play a role in the production of the chronic fatigue syndrome in genetically susceptible individuals. After a virus has infected the lymphocytes (cells of the immune system) they secrete a wide variety of chemicals including interferon, in order to fight the viral invasion. In the chronic fatigue syndrome it appears that this production of interferon may persist and be partially responsible for some of the symptoms.

In CFS there may be a disturbance in immune cell function. The mechanism which normally switches off the production of interferon seems to fail. Interferon is a naturally occurring chemical in the body which can also be synthesised in the laboratory and given by injection. It has been administered to patients with cancer, AIDS and other immunological disorders and of the noticeable side-effects severe fatigue is one of the most common. Other effects of excessive interferon or interferon treatment include headaches, musculo-skeletal pain, irritability, depression, slowing of the mental functions and fevers. Hence many of the symptoms of interferon excess mimic those of the chronic fatigue syndrome. Given intravenously the potent nervous system side-effects include changes in mood and memory. It is believed that the interferon acts on the hypothalamus and hippocampus in the brain. The interferon actually passes directly to the nerve cells of the central nervous system and binds onto receptors on the nerve cell surface called opiate receptors. These are the receptors which bind the opiates such as heroin, morphine and other opium-like chemicals. It is postulated that as a consequence of attaching to opiate receptors and stimulating these receptors on nerve cells that the tiring, fatiguing and sleepiness-like effects of morphine and other similar drugs is mimicked by the interferon.

Another interesting observation of the use of interferon clinically has been that it actually reduces the time required for an individual to fall into the rapid eye movement (REM) or dream stage of sleeping.

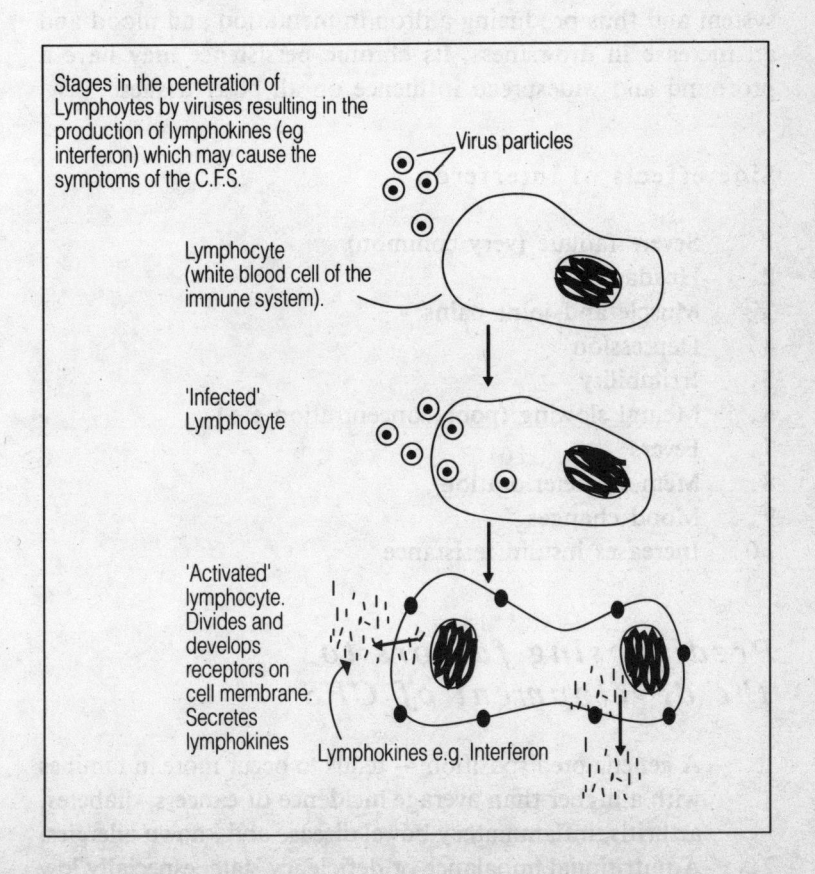

Stages in the penetration of Lymphoytes by viruses resulting in the production of lymphokines (eg interferon) which may cause the symptoms of the C.F.S.

Virus particles

Lymphocyte (white blood cell of the immune system).

'Infected' Lymphocyte

'Activated' lymphocyte. Divides and develops receptors on cell membrane. Secretes lymphokines

Lymphokines e.g. Interferon

Another possible harmful effect of interferon excess is that it increases the body's resistance to the effects of insulin. Insulin, in association with a chromium containing molecule called glucose tolerance factor, is essential for the transportation of glucose from the bloodstream into the cells of the body including the brain, liver, muscle cells and so on. If the action of insulin is inhibited by the presence of any factor including interferon, then the energy providing glucose molecules may not be presented in sufficient concentration to the body cells to maintain their optimal functioning. The role of chromium as a trace element is discussed elsewhere. Suffice to say here that very low chromium levels are not uncommon in CFS patients.

So while interferon in the short-term may play a beneficial role in an acute viral infection by slowing down the central nervous system and thus producing a drop in mentation and mood and an increase in drowsiness, its chronic persistence may have a profound and widespread influence on all body tissues.

Side effects of interferon

1. Severe fatigue (very common)
2. Headaches
3. Muscle and joint pains
4. Depression
5. Irritability
6. Mental slowing (poor concentration etc.)
7. Fevers
8. Memory deterioration
9. Mood changes
10. Increases insulin resistance

Predisposing factors to the development of CFS

1. A genetic predisposition — tends to occur more in families with a higher than average incidence of cancers, diabetes, arthritis, inflammatory bowel disease and known allergies.
2. A nutritional imbalance or deficiency state, especially low

levels of vitamin C, B-complex, zinc or selenium.
3. Chronic stress — emotional, physical, electromagnetic.
4. Chemical pollutants.
5. A viral or bacterial infection especially if poorly or incompletely resolved.
6. Antibiotic therapy.
7. Chronic bowel toxaemia from poor diet, junk food, poor food-combining.

Bacterial infections and the dangers of antibiotics

The majority of infectious diseases that present to doctors are caused by viral infections and these are generally self-limiting. However, over the past forty years there has been an increasing usage of antibiotics including the inappropriate prescribing of antibiotics for viral infections. Viruses are not susceptible to the killing actions of antibiotics and the use of preventative courses of antibiotics in case of secondary bacterial infections is generally not good medical practice.

The widespread prescription of antibiotics is regarded by microbiologists as potentially very dangerous. The development of resistant strains of bacteria to antibiotics is more likely the greater the exposure to these chemicals. However, even more sinister in the short-term are the effects that antibiotics have on the health of the individual. Antibiotics are synthetic or xenobiotic chemicals that require detoxification and place a load on the detoxifying mechanisms of the body. Because of their foreign nature, these antibiotics may also stimulate an allergic immune response to them. In doing so, these allergic reactions often spread to include other similar chemicals that appear in the food chain. Antibiotics are also known to induce liver enzymes and thus unnecessarily distress this organ.

Probably the most damaging effects of antibiotics — especially the broad spectrum type — are the destruction of the healthy microorganisms in the gastrointestinal tract and their subsequent replacement after antibiotic therapy ceases by potentially pathogenic bacteria and widespread infestation with the yeast, candida albicans.

Candida

Candidiasis is the condition caused by the yeast candida albicans which is an important disease causing microorganism. Candida is a well known cause of oral and vaginal thrush and sometimes infections of the skin where moisture occurs, for example, under the breasts, between the buttocks and between fatfolds. It is not so well known that candida can also cause death in people who have severely depressed immune function.

Candida occurs as a consequence of a weakening of the immune system, malnutrition, the use of antibiotics, the oral contraceptive pill, cortisone and chemotherapeutic drugs used in the treatment of cancer. Inadvertent exposure to antibiotics occurs in the general population through the consumption of poultry, pork and other meats grown with the use of antibiotics.

In patients with the chronic fatigue syndrome nearly 70% report the use of antibiotics for the treatment of an acute viral infection within the three months prior to the initial onset of their illness. Others have used antibiotics for the treatment of acne or other infections.

The majority of young women with the chronic fatigue syndrome report the use of oral contraceptives and vaginal thrush, and in many instances a previous history of severe vaginal thrush correlates with the onset of symptoms of the chronic fatigue syndrome. The common drugs such as cortisone may also be implicated.

It has been shown that over 80% of patients with the chronic fatigue syndrome have abnormalities in immune functioning, levels of antibodies, numbers of T-helper and T-depressor cells and allergy reactions. In fact, 90% of patients have moderate to high (significant) levels of IgE and IgG4 antibodies to specific candida antigens (proteins). These findings are suggestive that candida albicans is acting as an allergen and is chronically over-stimulating the immune system to function in an abnormal manner. Candida is also known to secrete a number of substances including acetaldehyde, a breakdown product of sugar and alcohol metabolism that causes the hangover effect the morning after a binge. These scientific findings are probably secondary to immune suppression caused primarily by the presence of heavy metals and xenobiotic chemicals.

Many symptoms are attributed to the presence of chronic candidiasis, some of which are non-specific and many of which are held in common with the chronic fatigue syndrome.

Most common symptoms of chronic candidiasis

1. Lethargy, fatigue, muscle weakness
2. Irritability, headaches or migraines
3. Muscle and joint pains
4. Irritable bowel syndrome
5. Sensitivity to yeast, alcohol and sugars
6. Cravings for sugar or alcohol
7. Cystitis without obvious infection
8. Anal or vaginal itching
9. Skin rashes that may appear like acne or psoriasis

The treatment of patients with candida albicans is very similar to the general treatment protocol for the management of the chronic fatigue syndrome outlined in Chapter 10. The basic principles of treatment are a diet that eliminates refined carbohydrates, for example, sugar, white flour products and alcohol and the elimination of yeast and fermented fruits from the diet. A reduction of total carbohydrate to approximately 60 grams per day is recommended and frequent snacks of protein foods are helpful. The absolute avoidance of drugs and medicines that promote the growth candida and other yeasts is mandatory. These drugs include antibiotics, cortisone, immunosuppressant drugs and the oral contraceptive pill. The avoidance of chicken and pork contaminated with antibiotics is also useful. Only free range eggs and chicken should be consumed.

A detoxification programme plus the use of immune supporting nutrients are generally required and the use of antifungal herbs, garlic, nystatin or ketoconazole may be needed. Nystatin and ketoconazole are both drugs but Nystatin is relatively safe. Ketoconazole has the potential for sometimes causing severe side effects to the chemically sensitive patients with the chronic fatigue syndrome and should only be used as a last resort. Lactobacillus and bifidobacteria are two micro-organisms that can be consumed orally in powder form and which have a suppressive effect on the overgrowth of yeasts and candida in the bowel and vagina. Their use is mandatory in the patient with diagnosed candidiasis.

CHAPTER FIVE

Chemicals, drugs and electromagnetic pollution

Case study

> John Birch, aged 28, thought that he was going to die. Shortly after dinner one night he suffered from an excruciating, heavy, crushing chest pain associated with severe shortness of breath and a 'sense of death'. He felt so weak that he could hardly move.
>
> He was immediately admitted to a major teaching hospital and investigated with blood tests, X-ray, CAT-scans and a cardiograph. To the surprise of his doctors all the tests returned negative. John became a medical dilemma. His symptoms persisted, continuing to get worse despite being seen by specialist physicians, neurologists and even a psychiatrist. It wasn't until one doctor took note of a special point in John's history that the cause of his problems became evident. Earlier in the day John, a spray painter, had been confined to an atmosphere containing a high concentration of paint fumes and solvents. Normally in such a situation he would wear a protective mask, but on this occasion he didn't. During the day he noticed one or two episodes of faintness and a fogginess in the head. The fumes

made him cough periodically but he disregarded these symptoms.

The doctor suspected a chemical induced sensitivity state. His condition continued to deteriorate until it was decided to commence a detoxification programme — the principle agent being vitamin C. Intravenous vitamin C (sodium ascorbate) was given in doses of 60 grams per day initially. Within the first couple of hours John's symptoms began to disappear and after 24 hours he was back to normal. However, it was necessary to continue intravenous vitamin C for a number of weeks until the effects of the solvents wore off.

The toxic chemical cocktail

Many of these chemical solvents that are used in industry and in the home have a high affinity for the lungs, nervous system, heart and brain and can be extremely destructive to these tissues.

The above case study is an example of an acute poisoning with a xenobiotic (synthetic) chemical. It is one of the more unusual methods by which poisoning occurs. The high levels of herbicide, pesticide, fungicide and other residues of chemicals in use today that are present in our air, food and water supply contribute to one of the most threatening problems in the history of the earth. All living things are exposed to these chemicals and almost without exception concentrations of these chemicals are slowly but surely building up in their tissues.

Pesticide residues have been found in animals living on the polar icecaps and in fact the residues themselves have been found a metre beneath the surface of the ice at the poles. Hundred of thousands of tonnes of these chemicals are produced annually and are indiscriminately sprayed over our lands and crops.

Major sources of body pollutants

1. Direct contact with chemicals at home and in the workplace.
2. Herbicide and pesticide residues from agricultural and veterinary chemicals.
3. Food metabolites resulting in biochemical sensitivity (sometimes incorrectly referred to as 'allergy')
4. Food contaminants including colourings, flavourings, preservatives, emulsifiers and other food additives.
5. Air and water pollutants including petrochemicals, chlorine and fluoride.
6. Heavy metal sources including mercury amalgam (dental fillings), lead, cadmium, arsenic, aluminium.
7. Bowel toxaemia including abnormal bowel flora (germs), candida and other yeasts, endotoxins, bacterial waste products.
8. Medicines, prescribed drugs and anaesthetics.

Bob's story

Severe drowsiness during the day was beginning to affect Bob's ability to stay awake at the wheel of his taxi. Bob was overweight and had been told by his doctor to lose weight because of the fear of heart disease which had plagued other family members.

Bob's blood pressure was elevated and he had been placed on a beta-blocking drug only a few months before. In his history, Bob had noticed that he became more tired after smoking and he had decided to quit. This did help his fatigue a little but not sufficiently to satisfy him. He also noticed that his fatigue and associated muscular weakness and aches and pains were worse during heavy smog days.

It appeared Bob was suffering from a chemical hypersensitivity syndrome, perhaps initiated by the beta-blocking drug for his blood pressure. Over the next few months his weight was reduced and his blood pressure medication changed. His fatigue lifted dramatically. After

> an overnight fast and a re-challenge with a very small dose of the initial beta-blocking drug, it was found that a profound sense of tiredness and fatigue developed.
>
> Bob's sensitivity to petrochemical smog also decreased after the principal cause of his chemical sensitivity had been found and eliminated.

This case illustrates the importance of finding the cause of a clinical condition and not just treating its symptoms. The discovery of the cause may begin with only a slight clinical suspicion as the only clue with which to start.

The heavy metals lead and mercury are discussed in Chapter 3 — *The Causes of Tiredness* as they are considered the prime causes for the development of susceptibility to the chronic fatigue syndrome.

In 1972 a study comparing the organochlorine residues in the body fat of people from eleven different nations revealed that Australians were found to have more than 2.5 times the level of dieldrin than in those from the other ten countries. Because Australia continues to use these organochlorine chemicals and other nations banned or severely restricted their use in the 1960s, we should expect that Australians would now have even higher concentrations than the rest of the world's population. In fact, recent studies have shown that levels of some of these organochlorine pesticide residues are three to ten times higher in Australian blood samples than in the average American. These chemicals include such things as dieldrin, DDT, DDE, DDD, hexachlorobenzene, xylene, benzene and chloroform.

Most of these toxic chemicals are stored in the body fat including the nerves and brain. It may take from three months to thirty years or longer for the levels of chemicals to be reduced to half their concentration in the body tissues after exposure to them has ceased. Over three million chemicals are listed on registers in the United States and more than 65,000 are in common use in the home, agriculture and industry. The vast majority of these chemicals were unknown before the second world war. So it can be seen that our exposure to this toxic chemical cocktail has only really occurred over the last fifty years. As a species, we are probably more polluted now than we have been at an other time in the history of humankind. **One may conclude from this that the exposure of living things to synthetic and potentially highly toxic chemicals is one of the greatest uncontrolled experiments ever designed on living things.**

Free radicals and chemical sensitivity

Chemicals can do damage to the body cells by a number of mechanisms. A sufficiently high enough dose of toxic chemicals will actually kill cells, but these are not the levels that we are concerned with here. Chronic low level exposures to chemicals that do not kill cells but effect their structure and functioning are the most common.

The most widespread damage done by these synthetic substances is via the mechanism of free radicals. Free radicals are molecules that have gained or lost an electric charge called an electron. An electron is a negatively charged particle that spins in orbit around atoms. For example, if a molecule of oxygen, which consists of two atoms of oxygen, gains an electron from an external source, it becomes negatively charged and therefore electrochemically unbalanced. This oxygen molecule with an extra electron is known as the superoxide radical. It is only one of possibly thousands of different radicals that can form in the body, others being hydroxyl radicals and peroxide radicals. These free radicals are very reactive molecules in that they can very rapidly transfer electrons from one source to another via themselves. In doing so, there is a very fast exchange of energy during these single electron transfers and this exchange of energy has the potential for doing a lot of good in the right place, and yet a lot of harm in others.

Free radicals are very short lived species of molecules and may last from millionths of a second to one or two seconds. Electron transfer, and therefore energy transfer, is very important in biological systems. Chemical stress to the living system occurs when toxic metabolites of various environmental chemicals interfere with this normal flow of electrons. There are many chemicals with the potential to produce free radicals both in the environment and within living cells themselves. The production of free radicals and other highly active molecular species can occur as a consequence of exposure not only to chemicals but to biological substances, radiation, sunlight and even by chance. Here we are mainly concerned with the types of chemicals that produce free radicals in biological systems. Free radical inducing chemicals are ubiquitous and have become a solemn, critical and urgent threat to mankind.

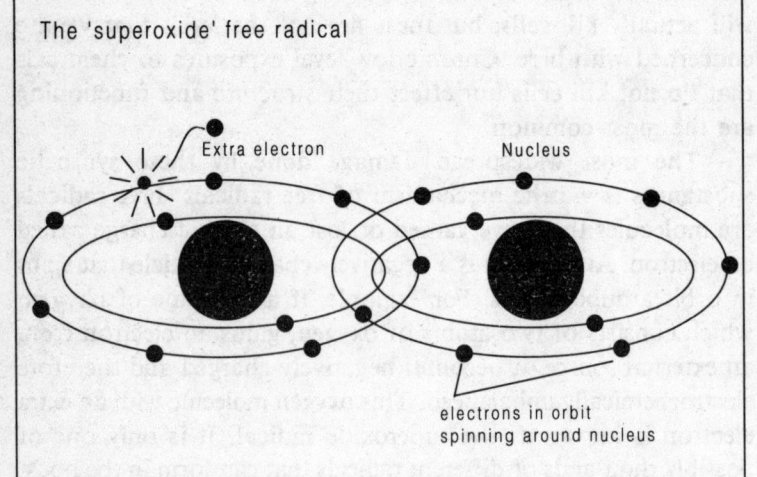

The 'superoxide' free radical

Extra electron — Nucleus

electrons in orbit spinning around nucleus

The oxygen molecule is made up of 2 nuclei surrounded by many electrons spinning around in their orbits. Thus the normal oxygen molecule is represented by the abbreviation (O_2).

When an extra electron is added to this system, it becomes (O_2)⁻ and it becomes electrochemically unbalanced and highly reactive.

A suitable antioxidant, for example ascorbic acid, will remove the electron and transfer it to an electron 'sink' (e.g. Vitamin E) where it is trapped and can cause no further damage.

Chemicals producing free radicals

1. Chlorinated hydrocarbons
2. Aromatic hydrocarbons
3. Industrial Acids and Solvents
4. Pesticides, herbicides and fungicides
5. Food preservatives and additives
6. Printing pigments and inks
7. Cosmetic vehicles
8. Fragrances and perfume vehicles
9. Air and water pollutants
10. Pharmacological agents and medical drugs
11. Anaesthetics
12. Ethanol (common alcohol found in beer, wine and spirits)

How do these free radicals damage the body cells, what do they do and what is the relationship to the chronic fatigue syndrome?

The answers to these and many other questions are important in that the proper management of the patient with the chronic fatigue syndrome is almost totally dependent on them. In fact, I have coined a new term for this molecular disease called Free Radical Disease.

Free radical disease

Free radical disease is defined as a disease of cellular and tissue destruction caused by free radical species as a consequence of the excessive production of free radical molecules in parts of the cells and tissues where they are not required and in which antioxidant capabilities have become relatively exhausted. (Brighthope, I.E., 1982.)

Radicals are produced in cells for necessary biological functions. For example, electron transfers occur constantly in the mitochondria where respiration and energy production occur. Oxidation of chemicals and metabolites is necessary as a part of normal biological function. The white blood cells of the body produce free radicals to destroy invading bacteria and viruses. Even our body's own hormones can be converted to free radicals as a part of their degradation processes and elimination in the body. For example, adrenalin and noradrenaline, the stress hormones, are converted by a process of auto-oxidation, to free radicals. An excessive production of these hormones under more stress than is required for normal living results in the production of excess free radicals. These may have the potential to cause biological degeneration, tissue damage and subsequent illness.

Larry's detoxification

> For 18 years nobody believed Larry. Aged 58 and a market gardener all his life, Larry felt more like 88. Eighteen years ago this very active man had been told by his employer to spray some weeds with DDT. While pouring the chemical into a container it splashed into his face. Immediately Larry noticed a painful burning sensation in the nose and mouth and the inhaled fumes started him coughing. For the next few weeks he felt generally unwell, with tiredness and muscle aches and pains being the major problems.
>
> His doctor told him that nothing was wrong and insisted that he return to work. Larry took a two week holiday by the sea and felt much better. He decided to return to work. Within a week, an employee was spraying a mixture of pesticides and the mist drifted in Larry's direction. Within minutes he started to choke, having chest pains and stomach cramps that he described as unbelievable.
>
> Following hospital admissions, many tests and many specialists, Larry was again told that nothing could be found. For the next 18 years Larry suffered — nobody believed him and he was chronically ill with severe fatigue, lethargy and depression. He was also very resentful of the medical profession for not 'listening' properly to his story.
>
> After 18 years of 'sheer hell' Larry visited a doctor specialising in nutritional and environmental medicine who performed some tests on his blood which showed high levels of DDT, DDE and DDD in his blood. Larry was also low in vitamin C and selenium and the detoxifying enzyme glutathione peroxidase. Larry was placed on a detoxifying diet, nutritional supplements and very high doses of selenium and vitamin C. His recovery was slow but sure.

His neurological functions markedly improved over the first three months and the improvement in his heart and lungs followed. An unfortunate chest infection occurred after five months which laid him up in hospital from 'pneumonia' from which he recovered exceedingly quickly. This was not an infection pneumonia but probably a chemical pneumonitis caused by the treatment mobilising the toxins that has accumulated in Larry's tissues over the previous 18 years.

This story is typical of the thousands of patients suffering from the chemical hypersensitivity syndrome mediated by free radical pathology.

Living cells are composed of an outer cell membrane and an internal nucleus that is responsible for the reproduction of the cell and its inherited features. Other structures within the cell include the golgi apparatus, the endoplasmic reticulum, lysomes and mitochondria. All of these are surrounded by membranes. The cell membranes, nuclear membrane and membranes lining the other intracellular components are very similar. They consist of a sandwich-like structure in which the pieces of bread are sheets of protein and the filling inside the sandwich are special lipids. The lipids inside these membranes consist of bonds that hold the atoms together. Some of these bonds are very susceptible to attack by free radicals. The bonds in the lipids can be virtually destroyed by free radicals in a very short time. As a consequence of this, the structure and therefore the functioning of these membranes is affected. It is at this level that we must consider protecting the molecules against free radical damage by the use of protective and buffering substances. These protective and buffering substances occur in nature and are commonly known as anti-free radical agents or antioxidants. A very well known antioxidant is present in the green leaves of plants to protect them against the harmful effects of radiation and radiation by-products (singlet-oxygen free radical). This substance is known as beta-carotene — the precursor to vitamin A.

We all live in a hostile environment. In fact, ever since living things existed, their environments have been to a large extent potentially lethal. Living cells need oxygen to help burn fuels (from food) to produce energy for life functions. Oxygen is a very reactive gas and by itself can cause spontaneous burning. To protect living cells against combustion and self destruction, antioxidants are necessary.

Probably one of the most hostile environments and situations for a human being is an intensive care unit. It is here that a patient with severe tissue damage, lacerations, fractured limbs, crushed chest and who is receiving intravenous drugs and chemicals and having oxygen delivered via a plastic tube to the airways is at greatest risk of oxidative damage to tissues and cells. The tissues damaged by trauma release very high levels of free radicals. The intravenous medications have the potential for producing more free radicals. The oxygen going into the lungs is another good source of oxidative damage. In this situation, the excessively high levels of oxidative free radicals place a load on the patient's antioxidant mechanisms and may even exhaust them. Should antioxidant levels in blood and tissues drop below a critical level, greater risks of complications and further degenerative disease is highly likely. Thus the ideal situation to study the effects of antioxidants in humans is in an intensive care situation or a burns unit.

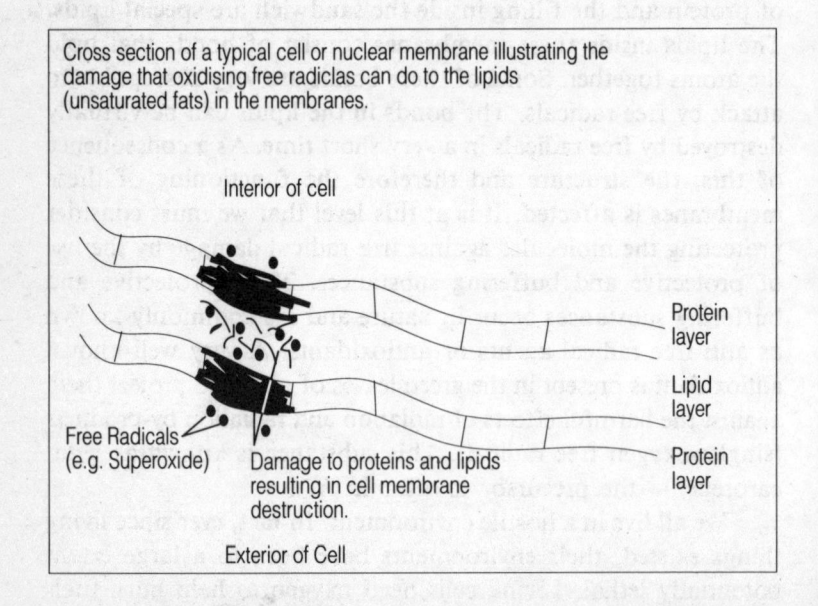

Cross section of a typical cell or nuclear membrane illustrating the damage that oxidising free radiclas can do to the lipids (unsaturated fats) in the membranes.

Interior of cell

Protein layer

Lipid layer

Free Radicals (e.g. Superoxide)

Damage to proteins and lipids resulting in cell membrane destruction.

Protein layer

Exterior of Cell

It was the oil chemists in the 1940s who first became aware of lipid peroxidation through oxidising free radicals. They discovered the activities of free radicals in the process of autocatalysis. Spectacular forms of chemical breakdown were observed in oils but it was not realised until decades later that similar chemical breakdowns occur in biological systems. We now know that the process of rancidity of foods is the result of a breakdown of fats and lipids, probably mediated through oxidative free radical attack. A biological example is the rancidification of butter. The naturally occurring antioxidants in butter continually mop up oxidising free radicals being produced in the fat. After a certain period of time the antioxidant mechanisms become totally saturated with free radicals and are unable to continue their antioxidant task. As a consequence, the butter goes rancid — that is, the molecular structure of its lipid molecules breaks down.

Many biological molecules including proteins, nuclear proteins in chromosomes and lipoproteins are subject to attack by free radicals. As a consequence of these attacks, there is fragmentation of the molecules with the production of what is termed Free Radical Oxidation Products (FROPS — first coined by I.E. Brighthope). These FROPS (Free Radical Oxidation Products) become increasingly water soluble the more they are broken down into smaller molecules. They have been found to be extraordinarily powerful in a wide range of biological systems. FROPS are potentially lethal. However, some fragments may have considerable survival value for the living cell and organism. FROPS have been shown to be cytotoxic to malignant cells and they are known to inhibit the replication of bacteria and viruses and even destroy bacteria outright. They are known to have an effect on the stickiness of the blood platelets and therefore play a role in the process of thrombosis or clotting of blood. Prostaglandins are a family of lipid-like substances that are also modulated by FROPS in their activity as anti-inflammatory and pro-inflammatory agents. However, the most interesting aspect of FROPS is that they have been shown to play a role in neuromuscular transmission.

Neuromuscular transmission is the transmission of impulses from the nerve to a muscle across a very narrow cleft. Messages from the brain which cause muscles to travel by electrochemical impulses down nerve fibres until they reach a muscle cell. Small packets of chemicals are released at the end of the nerve fibre and travel to the membrane of the muscle cell. When these chemicals, called neurotransmitters, reach the muscle cell membrane they initiate a series of chemical reactions which change the electricity inside the cell and the muscle cell thereby contracts, creating movement. Free radicals have been shown to influence this neuromuscular transmission between the nerve fibre and the muscle cell.

It could be that a number of possible mechanisms exist for transmission disturbances to occur in the patient with the chronic fatigue syndrome. Firstly, free radicals may interfere with the release of the chemical messages from the end of the nerve fibre. Secondly, free radicals themselves may act as false neurotransmitters and block the effect of the true neurotransmitters at the muscle cell membrane, thereby preventing it contracting. Thirdly, the free radicals themselves may bind onto the muscle cell membrane and interfere with its reception of the neurotransmitters. Fourthly, the free radicals themselves may damage the cell membrane and intracellular structures of muscle cells.

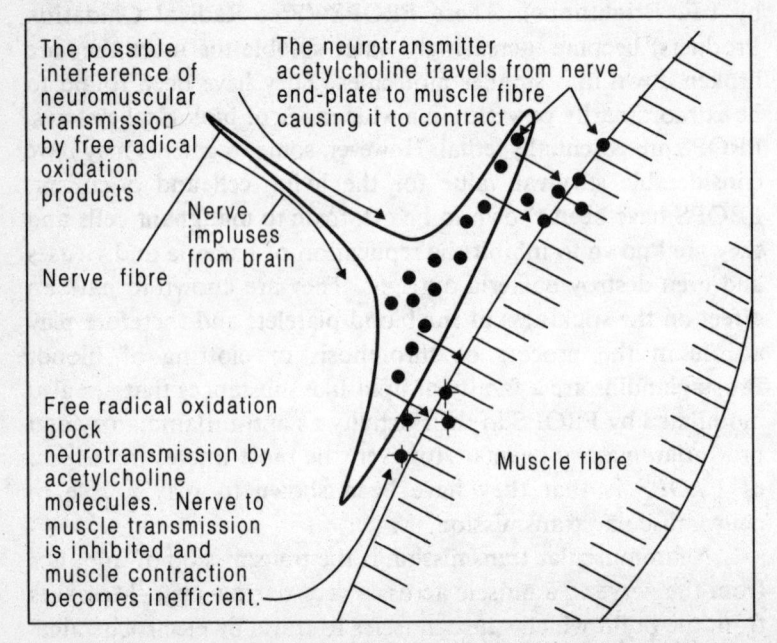

The possible interference of neuromuscular transmission by free radical oxidation products

The neurotransmitter acetylcholine travels from nerve end-plate to muscle fibre causing it to contract

Nerve impulses from brain

Nerve fibre

Free radical oxidation block neurotransmission by acetylcholine molecules. Nerve to muscle transmission is inhibited and muscle contraction becomes inefficient.

Muscle fibre

At present there is only indirect clinical evidence that this is occurring in the chronic fatigue syndrome and more research is required. However, all the evidence available to-date points to this syndrome as being a manifestation of, for want of a better term, free radical disease.

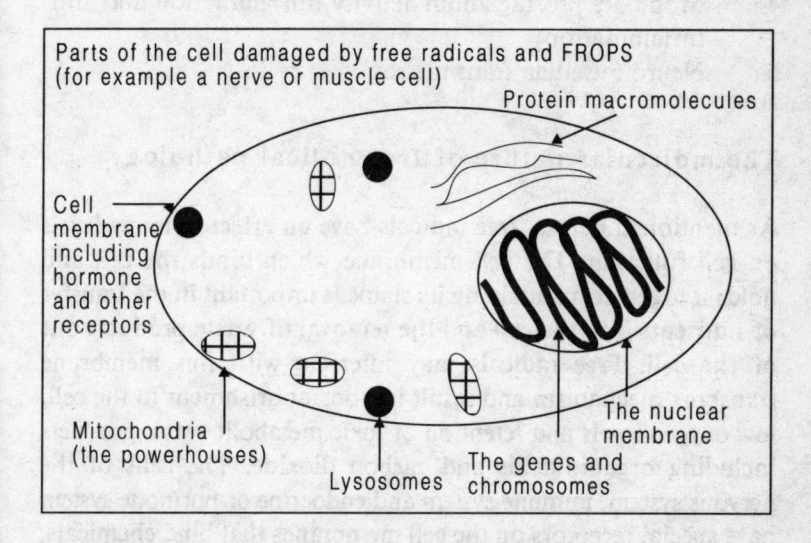

Parts of the cell damaged by free radicals and FROPS (for example a nerve or muscle cell)

- Protein macromolecules
- Cell membrane including hormone and other receptors
- Mitochondria (the powerhouses)
- Lysosomes
- The genes and chromosomes
- The nuclear membrane

Factors causing chemical mobilisation

1. Lactation
2. Exercise
3. Fever
4. Infections
5. Fasting
6. Severe emotional stress
7. Nutritional deficiencies

Effects of chemical mobilisation

1. Immune damage
2. Nerve damage
3. Endocrine (hormonal) damage

The actions of FROPS — Free radical oxidation products

1. Toxic to malignant cells
2. Inhibit or kill bacteria and viruses
3. Influence the stickiness of blood platelets (bleeding and clotting)
4. Modulate prostaglandin activity (inflammation and anti-inflammation)
5. Neuromuscular transmission

The molecular nature of free radical pathology

As mentioned before, free radicals have an effect at many levels on cell function. The cell membrane which binds the cell and holds it together maintaining its shape is important in the transfer of nutrients into the cell and the removal of waste products out of the cell. Free radicals may interfere with this membrane transport mechanism and result in poor nourishment to the cell, low oxygen levels and retention of toxic metabolic waste products including organic acids and carbon dioxide. The cells of the nervous system, immune system and endocrine or hormone system have special receptors on the cell membranes that bind chemicals, for example hormones and neurotransmitters. This binding is necessary in order that the chemical transmitter can do its work and make the cell function in a particular way.

Damage to these surface receptors by free radicals can change their three dimensional structure to such a degree that the hormone for example, will no longer bind to the cell. Furthermore, if the membrane is damaged severely enough by the free radical attack, valuable metabolites may actually leak from the cell which may eventually result in cell death. Another mechanism by which cells can be damaged by free radicals is through the disruption of lysosomes within the cell itself. Lysosomes are small bodies bound by membranes and they contain very potent enzymes for the destruction of bacteria and viruses when they enter the cell. An excessive or inappropriate release of these enzymes by free radical attack on lysosomal membranes may result in gross intracellular damage and possibly death.

Prostanoids are hormone-like substances that are made from the essential fatty acids in the diet. These prostanoids are involved in the production of inflammation for tissue repair, the production of anti-inflammatory agents, the dilation and/or constriction of blood vessels and airways and the initiation and/or inhibition of the coagulation of the blood. Hence prostanoids play an extremely important role in many physiological processes throughout the body. The synthesis of these very potent prostanoid substances which include prostaglandins, leucotrienes, thromboxane and platelet activating factor is influenced by the presence of free radical molecules. This may result in an enhanced or exaggerated inflammatory response, an increase in the tendency of blood to coagulate and form thrombosis or an excessive constriction of blood vessels or narrowing of airways in the lung.

Many of the manifestations of allergies are mediated through the effects of these prostanoid substances. In fact at the molecular level, free radicals influence the cells of the immune system in a number of ways including altering the antigens on the surface of the immune cell membranes and also changing the nature of antibody receptors. The presence of high levels of free radicals is also associated with changes in the white blood cells including a reduction in helper cells, suppressor cells and natural killer cells, thus affecting efficiency and effectiveness of the entire immune system. To protect and buffer the various structures of the living cell against free radical attack, living things must maintain a constant antioxidant potential. This can be achieved with suitable natural-occurring antioxidants.

Antioxidant mechanisms present in nature

In the discussion on free radical disease and the effects of free radicals on biological systems, the study of antioxidant mechanisms that occur in nature is mandatory. These mechanisms involve the use of naturally occurring substances that combine to collect or mop up free radicals or act as a sink for the storage of unbridled electrons. Antioxidant mechanisms include proteins present in the bloodstream such as the copper-containing caeruloplasmin or the iron transporting protein transferrin.

Caeruloplasmin is one of the most potent inhibitors of free

radicals and it is extremely active immediately after tissue has been injured or damaged. On the other hand, transferrin is a protein that binds iron. It is known that free iron in the tissues actually catalyses the production of free radical oxidation reactions. The binding of iron to transferrin by chelation prevents these harmful reactions occurring. Antioxidant enzymes also exist in every cell of the body for protection against free radicals. These enzymes include superoxide dismutase (SOD), glutathione peroxidase and catalase. Superoxide dismutase deactivates superoxide free radicals and is dependent on an adequate supply of zinc, manganese or copper. Glutathione peroxidase is an enzyme that inactivates peroxides. These are also very reactive chemicals and glutathione peroxidase is dependent on the trace element selenium for its functioning.

An adequate supply of these trace elements and micronutrients is therefore important for the normal functioning of these protective and detoxifying enzyme systems. Other nutrients are also required for the optimal functioning of glutathione peroxidase, such as methionine and vitamin C. Glutathione peroxidase is important as a naturally occurring anti-inflammatory enzyme, for the production of antibodies and for protection against cancer. The activity of glutathione peroxidase is reduced by toxic chemical overload, fasting and selenium deficiency states.

Patients with the chronic fatigue syndrome who are known to be sensitive to chemicals show either a very low level of selenium in their blood or a diminished activity of this glutathione peroxidase. As the name suggests, the enzyme glutathione peroxidase also requires an adequate supply of glutathione, a molecule containing three amino acids and sulphur. To fuel the production of this glutathione we need an adequate supply of a critical antioxidant called NADH. NADH stands for reduced nicotinamide adenine dinucleotide and its presence and activity is determined by the level of niacin or vitamin B3 in the diet.

It can therefore be seen that there is a noticeable interdependence between these active substances and nutrients.

Probably the most important nutrients acting as nutrients in the critical antioxidant process are vitamins A (beta-carotene), C (ascorbic acid) and E (tocopherol). Beta-carotene has been mentioned before as an important antioxidant in its mechanisms of squelching singlet-oxygen. Singlet-oxygen is a single oxygen atom which can act as a free radical promoter. The most important antioxidant in the water soluble compartments of the cells and tissues, is ascorbic acid. It is the prime free radical scavenger.

Ascorbic acid is discussed in great detail in Chapter 7 and as a single therapeutic substance it represents the most effective treatment modality for patients with the chronic fatigue syndrome that has been used to-date and probably in the future.

Vitamin E or tocopherol is a fat soluble substance that acts as a sink for free radicals in the fatty tissues and lipid molecules of the body. It is also discussed in more detail in Chapter 7.

An important message here is that while these antioxidant substances and mechanisms are given various names, they do not act independently of one another. Free radicals are inactivated when one antioxidant molecule accepts a negatively charged electron from the free radical and neutralises it. The antioxidant then has to do something with the charged electron and it either buries it deep inside its molecular structure or it passes it on to another antioxidant molecule which may pass it on to others until such time as the appropriate mopping up or expulsion can be performed.

Antioxidant mechanisms in nature

1. Caeruloplasmin (copper containing protein)
2. Transferrin (iron containing protein)
3. Antioxidant enzymes (superoxide dismutase, glutathione peroxidase, catalase)
4. Trace elements (zinc, copper, manganese, selenium)
5. Vitamins (beta-carotene, ascorbic acid, tocopherol)
6. Bioflavonoids

In the study of the major pathological processes that occur in disease, it has become more evident over recent years that free radicals play a role, perhaps even the major role, in the production of these processes. The four main pathological processes are inflammation, carcinogenesis (cancer promotion), thrombosis (blood clotting) and hypoxic tissue damage (damage in tissues due to a lack of blood supply).

Scientific studies have shown that virtually all of the antioxidants have an anti-inflammatory effect. Deficiencies of some antioxidants are associated with carcinogenesis and some have even been demonstrated to block the formation of carcinogenic substances. For example, nitrites in the diet are converted in the intestines to carcinogenic nitrosamines. This conversion is blocked by the presence of ascorbic acid (vitamin C). Most of the antioxidants have also been shown to be deficient in blood clotting disorders and thrombosis and some, for example vitamins E and C, can actually reduce the thrombotic tendency.

Finally, it has been extremely well demonstrated in animal studies that adequate tissue levels of antioxidants will protect that tissue against hypoxic damage when the blood supply is temporarily cut off. This has important implications in diseases such as atherosclerosis, coronary heart disease and stroke.

What significance does this all have for the patient with the chronic fatigue syndrome?

If one examines the signs and symptoms of deficiencies of most of these antioxidant nutrients, the common and often most prominent symptom throughout is fatigue or tiredness and lethargy. In the chronic fatigue syndrome patient, it is not simply the deficiency of a particular nutrient but a combination of factors including normal but very low levels of antioxidants, higher than average levels of heavy metals and an increased susceptibility to sensitivity to foods, chemicals and possibly free radicals that are responsible for the syndrome.

Life has evolved along interfaces between lipids and nonlipids and in fact it is a wonderful creation in immisçible media. The unsaturated lipids in the cells of the body are drenched with oxygen — the energy giving gas that in particular situations causes untold oxidative damage. Suitable antioxidants reside in healthy living tissues. Antioxidant protection in the living is a function of these substances and of structural integrity. Damaged cells loose structural integrity and are subject to free radical damage. This of course is the mechanism by which they are destroyed and removed to be replaced in some tissues by newly formed cells.

Irreversibly damaged cells don't merely disintegrate. They are like the fuel tanks of crashing planes - they explode with free radical release and damage occurring locally and then spreading if antioxidant defence capabilities are low or have been compromised. Thus tissue damage due to a virus, bacteria, yeast, trauma, chemicals, radiation etc. may not be restricted to local short-term degeneration but it may contribute to the propagation of radical-mediated disease at a distance to the primary site.

These molecular events most definitely play a role in the chronic fatigue syndrome — the question remains, to exactly what extent?

Diseases proven to be caused by pesticides and herbicides

1. Spina bifida
2. Cleft palate
3. Specific cancers
4. Spontaneous abortion
5. Increased neonatal deaths
6. Renal agenesis (failure of kidneys to develop in the foetus)

The sources of household chemicals

1. All detergents
2. Soft vinyl furniture
3. Synthetic bedding
4. Polyester clothing
5. Cheap paints — give off gases
6. Foam upholstery
7. Synthetic carpets
8. Cleaning sprays and materials
9. Hair sprays
10. Cosmetics, soaps, toothpaste
11. Gas heaters
12. Air-conditioning units
13. Plastics (including plastic furniture) — nearly all plastics emit gases

14. Newsprint
15. Vaporising bitumen

The 'sick building' syndrome

1. Modern buildings are almost completely sealed units
2. Concentration of gaseous chemicals e.g. formaldehyde produced from urea foam insulation, off-gassing plastics, toluene, benzene, xylene, natural gas etc.
3. Improvements made by increased ventilation and filtration of air, negative ionization of air, full natural spectrum light and the use of fewer off-gassing synthetics

Chemicals found in high concentrations in the blood of Australian sufferers of chronic fatigue syndrome

1. Organochlorines
2. Styrene and xylene
3. Chloroform
4. Trichloroethane
5. Tetrachloroethylene

Xenobiotic transformation

One of the frightening aspects of the chemicals polluting our environment is that of the possibility of xenobiotic transformation. This is a change in the chemical's structure that may occur to any number of synthetic chemicals which results in a more potent or toxic substance.

Recently it has been discovered that bacteria lying on the beds of the Mississippi in the United States have the ability to convert organochlorine chemicals into different substances. It has generally been believed that this biological transformation results in a less toxic molecule. However, this is not necessarily the case. In fact, some biochemists have shown that the enzyme systems in our own bodies have the ability to combine different pesticides and herbicides into compounds that resemble the deadly nerve gases used in chemical warfare.

It is possible that small quantities of nerve toxins are being constantly produced in the patients with the chronic fatigue syndrome, especially in those patients who have exceedingly high levels of these pesticide and herbicide residues. Unfortunately, very little good research is being performed in these areas and toxicologists, probably for political and financial reasons, are not addressing the problems satisfactorily.

Lethal synergism

Toxicology, or the study of the toxic effects of poisons and noxious substances on living tissues, is an extremely crude and inexact science. For example, a chemical substance tested in animals and shown not to produce disease in a relatively short time, is often regarded as safe and therefore able to be used in the broader community. These short-term animal studies do not take into consideration a number of factors including the effects of long-term exposure, the cumulative effects of toxic substances in the body and — probably most important of all — the synergistic effect between the tested chemical and thousands of other chemicals present in the environment.

It has been demonstrated in partridges for example that a lethal synergism exists between two chemicals, either of which when used individually are safe but when combined can cause death in these birds.

With over 60,000 xenobiotic synthetic chemicals in use, the number of synergistic combinations is almost infinite. Toxicology does not take into account the effect of this synergism on the **health** of the animal or human being. It is only concerned with the production of **disease** by single chemicals.

Some facts on pesticides and herbicides

1. They definitely cause disease
2. Aerial spraying may result in 70% drift of the total application

3. Pesticide drifts may occur for hundreds perhaps thousands of miles
4. Evaporation of sprayed pesticides can range from 50% to 90%
5. Personnel using these sprays are generally untrained or inadequately trained

The chemicals

The general term pesticide refers to and includes such things as fungicides, insecticides, rodenticides (to kill rodents) and acaricides (to kill ticks, spiders and mice).

Sensitisation to any of these chemicals depends on the total chemical load on the individual and that load exceeding the individuals actual tolerance level to chemicals, either due to a massive and sudden acute exposure to chemicals or to a chronic cumulative effect.

Sensitisation to chemicals and/or their metabolites is also a consequence of synergism between chemicals and possibly also the alteration of the chemical structure by micro-organisms in the bowel and enzyme action in the liver. Once a person is sensitised to a chemical they may show an adverse reaction including a multitude of symptoms to a chemical that is considered relatively safe for the general population. A person's tolerance level for chemicals is related to their general health, genetic factors, state of nutrition, antioxidant status, degree of emotional stress, biochemical individuality and past medical history with particular reference to diseases of the nervous system, immune system and endocrine glands.

Malcolm's pre-senile dementia

> Tina and her husband Malcolm come from the Riverina district of New South Wales and they have lived there all their lives. They ran a rice farm and had been quite successful.
> But for three years Tina had supported Malcolm in his temper outbursts and tiredness. It became too much for her

when he started to forget simple but important things like collecting the children from school or turning on the oven for dinner. Following a referral to a specialist physician — who couldn't find anything wrong — and a psychiatrist — who said Malcolm was depressed — Tina sought the help of a neurologist who diagnosed possible pre-senile dementia. For the next six months life was in limbo for Tina. She had a family which she loved and a husband who was deteriorating in personality, mood and intellect. She returned to the neurologist who then sought another opinion. The second neurological opinion confirmed her worst fears — pre-senile dementia. Malcolm would soon be bedridden. But Tina was a fighter and wondered if there was something outside of orthodox medicine that could help. Browsing through her local health food shop one day she picked up a book titled *Nutrients to Age Without Senility* by a Canadian Professor of Psychiatry and MD. She learned that many people in the early stages of senility had been helped by this man and his colleagues. She decided to contact him and he advised Tina to contact the Orthomolecular Medical Association of Australia because he had associates in that organisation who would treat Malcolm in the manner he used in Canada. Although warned that the condition may be irreversible, Tina took her husband to Melbourne where he was diagnosed as having a vitamin B3 and zinc deficiency, probably caused by his chronic exposure to herbicide and pesticide sprays.

Like most rice farmers, Malcolm had been told by chemical salesmen that to increase crop yields, sprays must be used. In fact, for every crop he planted Malcolm applied over 20 applications of chemicals. Some cereal growers have learned that this is not necessary and that by using better crop management techniques, no synthetic chemicals are required.

Malcolm was given treatment very similar to that outlined at the end of this book and within six months he was back to normal, holidaying in Europe with his devoted family. From time to time he noticed his energy levels dropping off and this was easily corrected with a therapeutic dose of vitamin B3 250mg three times a day plus some B complex. Malcolm's nutritional medicine specialist advised him that to stay well he must continue with this programme for life because he had developed a vitamin dependent disorder — Malcolm was only too happy to do so.

Chlorinated hydrocarbons

These are pesticides that contain chlorine and they enter the body by ingestion of contaminated water, the inhalation of dusts, vapours and by skin contact. They include aldrin and dieldrin (which have now been banned in agriculture but are used for the treatment of termites), chlordane, heptachlor, DDT, DDE, DDD, endrin, hexachlorobenzene (HCB) and lindane.

All of these chemicals affect the nervous system and block the transmission of nerve impulses. The side effects of exposure include nausea, dizziness, tremors, muscle weakness, fatigue, excitability, nervous apprehension, disorientation and, if severe enough, convulsions and coma. They have a very long half life and are released from the fat stores in the body periodically during illness and other stress conditions.

Organophosphates

These are very cheap and widely used compounds that are also very persistent. They enter the body by inhalation, ingestion and absorbtion through the skin. They have a short half life and are not easily detected in blood. The organic phosphate compounds inhibit the activity of the enzyme, cholinesterase.

Cholinesterase is important for the breakdown of acetylcholine, which is an important neurotransmitter. An excess of this can cause what is known as a cholinergic crisis including nausea, vomiting, sweating, excessive salivation, tear production, blurring of vision, involuntary urination and defecation. Other problems of organophosphates include abnormal heart rhythms, asthma, mucous production, rapid heart rates, high blood pressure, muscle cramps and weakness, shortness of breath and, if severe, bronchitis, respiratory failure and paralysis.

Parathion is a member of this family and because of its toxicity has caused many deaths after exposure to dust and aerosols. Other members of this family include malathion, diazinon (highly toxic), dimethoate (rogor), dichlorvos (Shelltox strips) and demeton (systex).

The volatile chemicals

This is a large family of chemicals containing both halogenated and non-halogenated chemicals. Halogens are chemicals containing chlorine, bromine or fluorine in their molecular structure.

This family of chemicals contains solvents that are used in glues, adhesives, paint thinners, solvents for colouring, detergent, hundreds of synthetics, anaesthetics, petrol additives, refrigerants, fungicides, fire extinguishers, the dye industry, rodenticides and volatile aromatics used in thousands of industrial processes and consumer products. Examples are cyclopentane, hexane, pentane, benzene (toxic to brain and blood), toluene (used in glue sniffing — permanent brain damage), xylene, trimethyl-benzene (asthma and chemical lung damage), styrene, chloroform, trichloroethane, bromobenzene, ethylbromide, vinylbromide and so on.

The harmful effects of these chemicals include muscle fatigue, lethargy, psychological depression, headaches, sleepiness, pins and needles and numbness of the limbs, behaviour disorders, learning problems and respiratory problems including asthma, bronchitis and respiratory failure, irritations of the skin, mouth, nose and lungs, liver damage, hepatitis, bone marrow and blood disturbances, kidney damage, chromosomal breakage (possible genetic and carcinogenic effects) and even addiction, evidenced by the habit of glue sniffing using the volatile aromatic toluene (methylbenzene).

The phenols

These includes the chlorophenols, the PCBs, 2-4-D, 2-4-5-T, Agent Orange, dioxin (an impurity of 2-4-5-T) and paraquot (diquot). Again, these chemicals have wide use in agriculture, industry and the home and some are so toxic that they have been banned. The PCB subgroup are extremely dangerous having a high fat solubility and easy accumulation in the body tissue. They are very stable chemicals and primarily affect the enzymes responsible for respiration in the mitochondria of the cell. They are also known to deplete vitamin levels in the blood and liver. Again, side effects mimic those of the chronic fatigue syndrome.

The carbamate family

These are pesticides that are mainly derived from carbamic acid, a compound containing nitrogen that has a similar effect to the organophosphate family. They include carbaryl (sevin), aminocarb (matacil), and propoxur (Baygon).

These are the main families of chemicals that are used as pesticides but the list of individual chemicals within each family is even more extensive. There are many others but basically they all have similar effects on biological systems and they are all required to go through the detoxification process and pathways. If these detoxification pathways are inhibited or overloaded with chemicals, then somewhere along the process a bottleneck will occur resulting in a build up of chemicals and their metabolites. This results in increasing toxic load with the subsequent deterioration in health of the individual.

Eventually a cascade effect results with an increase in the number and severity of symptoms. In clinical practice a 'Spreading Phenomenon' occurs in which the patient eventually reacts to more and more chemicals at lower and lower concentrations.

Pesticide misuse

There are hundreds, perhaps thousands, of examples of gross chemical misuse and negligence that can be cited throughout Australia.

A report, prepared by the New South Wales Department of Agriculture was withheld from the public for over 18 months. This report contained the results of a survey of farmers in the Sydney region and it revealed that an alarming proportion of

vegetable and fruit growers were regularly misusing pesticides and putting themselves, their family, neighbours and the public at great risk. The most disturbing findings of the report were:
- It was found that one third of farmers didn't use any protective clothing when mixing and spraying pesticides and only one third of farmers actually had the correct safety equipment to apply them.
- Only a quarter of the farmers using pesticides actually understood the basic terminology of safe pesticide usage and over 50% actually sprayed pesticides under adverse weather conditions including high temperatures and winds (both contributing to pesticide evaporation and drift).

Hundreds of thousands of tonnes of these substances are used annually in agriculture and should be the cause of great concern to those using them, the public generally and authorities in the departments of health and agriculture.

Information about agricultural chemicals

1. Unsafe levels of pesticide residues occur in our food, water and air supply.
2. Levels of dieldrin found in human autopsies have been shown to be as high as twenty-two times that which is allowed in beef exports.
3. It has been stated that the levels of pesticide residues in Australians are so high that the fat would not have been fit for human consumption if we were cannibals (i.e. 'humans are not fit for export').
4. Chlordane is applied to the soil before concrete slaps are laid in housing. A thirty square house can sit on an application of four hundred gallons of this chemical. Pesticides used in household spraying have been detected in breast milk in nursing mothers living in sprayed homes. A level of one part per million pesticide in breast milk may rise to over seventy parts per million three weeks after spraying.
5. Malathion is an organophosphate used in the treatment of head lice (malathion is a known carcinogen).

6. If one part per million of dieldrin is detected in blood, five parts per million will be present in the brain, twenty-six parts per million will be present in the liver and over one hundred and fifty parts per million will be present in fatty tissue.
7. Scientific residue surveys in Australia to-date have been badly carried out.
8. Of over 24,000 samples recently examined, most were from meat and gain foodstuffs for export, and only 750 were from domestic fruit and vegetables.
9. Chemicals banned in the United States are still permitted in Australia (dieldrin).
10. Gross negligence concerning high residue levels in Australians has been documented again the public health authorities in Australia.
11. Residue levels in some Australians are ten times higher than the US average.
12. Australian government committees have so far failed to achieve necessary reforms.
13. The chemical industry has applied undue pressure on pesticide officers and bureaucrats of the various agriculture departments.
14. Australian figures on human pesticide poisonings are not available — inadequate record-keeping.
15. Chemicals that are banned or restricted overseas include dieldrin, eldrin, chlordane, heptachlor, dichlorvos, dimenthanoate and endosulfan.
16. Public health authorities in Australia do not take the hazards posed by carcinogenic or mutagenic substances sufficiently seriously.
17. The chemicals associations are very strong and well-financed lobbies who deal very effectively with a poorly educated and timid bureaucracy.
18. Over 40,000 fatal and non-fatal human pesticide poisonings occur annually in the United States — no accurate figures for Australia.
19. There is no safe level for a carcinogen.
20. Patients who have avoided chemicals and who use organically grown foods have achieved marked improvements in their health and sometimes the disappearance

of disease conditions.
21. Residues cause disease including spontaneous abortion, birth abnormalities, infertility, cancer, allergies, asthma, mental illness and contribute to most human degenerative disease.
22. The fact that chemicals are presumed innocent until proven guilty is testimony to the failure of science and infers possible scientific fraud.
23. The National Health and Medical Research Council's expertise in the assessment of chronic poisoning is seriously questionable.
24. The National Health and Medical Research Council has stated that there is very little research into whether chemicals do cause health problems because 'there is little evidence that they do'. This is a logical nonsense.
25. The NH&MRC believe that there is a great injustice being done to the community by informing them of the hazards of pesticide residues.
26. The medical profession generally does not consider chemicals as a cause of health problems in the majority if not all of their patients.
27. Spokespersons for the Anti-cancer Council of Victoria have stated that the risk of cancer related to chemicals used in the production or processing of food is virtually negligent. The degree of concern in the community is not justified by the evidence, 'so they' believe.
28. While medical and scientific authorities may appear quite rational in arguing the case for the safety of pesticides and herbicides their credibility is undermined with the evidence against these substances.
29. The world human population has increased as a partial consequence of the use of chemical pesticides and fertilisers providing more food. Inevitably, almost total dependence on the chemical industry will result. There may be no turning back.

Beware of officialdom

Twelve months prior to the world's top scientists cautioning us on the harmful climatic affects of the depletion of the ozone layer, global warming and other effects of global pollution, Australia's foremost meteorologists emphatically denied that climatic changes had or were about to occur. Similarly, in October 1989 in an article published in **The Bulletin**, the Chairman of the Australasian Association of Cancer Registries and Director of the Cancer Registry at the Anti-cancer Council of Victoria, stated that 'the public perception that pesticides and chemicals caused cancer and a range of other ills from birth defects to senility was wrong.' He went on to state that 'fears about cancer were not unfounded in a country where one person in three is likely to contract a form of cancer, but much of this anxiety has been caused by the media as a result of events such as the Agent Orange Royal Commission.' Six months after this statement the Agent Orange World Commission's findings were proven wrong.

So much for our reliance on science, technology and experts in positions of authority. The lesson here is to always doubt and always question.

Electromagnetic pollution (electromagnetic smog)

Before the discovery and use of electricity and electromagnetic forces, living things were exposed to electromagnetic influences generated by the earth and the sun. Since the advent of electricity and the subsequent use of power via high tension electric lines, electric motors, generators and the production of radio and television waves, the atmosphere has become a medium for the carriage of an enormous number of electromagnetic signals. Science and medicine have yet to define whether or not these signals affect the health and well-being of living things. The possibility of them causing disease has only been considered in recent years.

Some scientific workers believe that living near high tension overhead power lines results in an increase in some forms of leukaemia and others believe that siting houses over underground rivers may result in some forms of cancer. A higher incidence of suicide has been documented in populations living in close proximity to overhead power lines. It certainly makes sense to the person in the street that these electromagnetic forces from power lines may have an effect on health.

This belief is supported by the simple exercise of standing under power lines with a fluorescent tube in one hand and observing the spontaneous lighting of the tube.

Approximately one patient in five with the chronic fatigue syndrome can relate almost immediately the onset of fatigue when they come in close contact with radiation from TV sets, computer tubes, electric typewriters, hairdryers and even electric blankets. The radiation from TV sets and computers can produce a profound tiredness in some very sensitive individuals. It is interesting to note that in submarines, it was the seamen who operated the radar who suffered from most illness. The microwaves that were emitted by the radar screens actually caused the crazy seaman syndrome.

Patients with the chronic fatigue syndrome who may be sensitive to electromagnetic radiation should firstly avoid it as much as possible, occupy parts of the home and workplace away from power lines including those that are hidden, and they should attempt to earth themselves from time to time. This can be achieved simply by walking on the ground with bare feet, or by touching a water pipe that passes to the earth. Some natural therapists are recommending the use of special magnets and electronic brain tuning devices both of which are of benefit to electromagnetically sensitive fatigue patients.

CHAPTER SIX

Food and chemical sensitivity

Case study

> 'I discovered the damage that food could do to me 45 years ago when I was 20 and the eczema that I suffered throughout my childhood and adolescence disappeared after I stopped drinking milk on the advice of a friend,' said 65 year old William Tyson. 'By the time I was 25 I had "outgrown" my allergies according to my doctor and I started to use dairy products again. Within six months, I was getting migraine and skin rashes, both of which ended abruptly after I eliminated the dairy foods. Since I turned 60, I had been virtually crippled from arthritis and pain in the hands, shoulders, back and knees and the past five years have been sheer hell. Why I didn't suspect that my allergic tendency was causing this I don't know, but my wife recently suggested removing wheat, tomatoes and potatoes from my diet and miraculously, the pain and stiffness went almost overnight.'

William Tyson is one of approximately three million Australians who suffer from severe sensitivities to foods and/or chemicals. These sensitivities are often mistakenly labelled 'allergies', but less than 10% of them are allergies in the true sense. An allergy occurs as the result of a reaction in the blood between an ingested 'allergen' (e.g. milk protein, egg white, oranges) and an antibody formed by the immune system. On the other hand, a food or chemical sensitivity is an abnormal biochemical reaction in the body following exposure. There are hundreds, possibly thousands, of abnormal biochemical reactions that can occur and diagnosis of food/chemical sensitivity can be very difficult. In the case of Bill Tyson, the diagnosis was quite simple and it was made easier because his eczema was caused by one food only — milk. Had he not been made aware of this association between symptoms and food in his 20's, Bill may have continued to suffer from arthritis in later life until the day he died. The term food allergy in the rest of this article also includes food sensitivity.

Food allergy affects all of us from time to time and it is worse when we are under emotional or psychological stress. In fact, psychological stress symptoms may also occur as a result of food allergies (some doctors now refer to this as 'Brain Allergy') which in turn become amplified because of the stress.

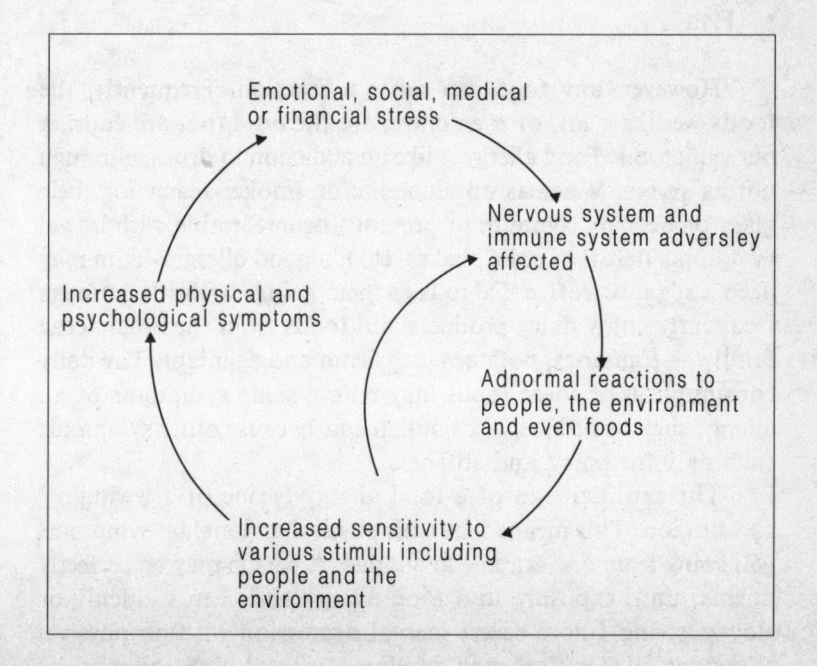

As the above diagram illustrates, a vicious cycle is created and the allergies become more frequent and severe as time, and stress, goes on.

Most people don't associate their frequent symptoms with allergy but in fact the symptoms of most diseases may be caused or aggravated by foods and chemicals. For example, it has been scientifically shown that pain, migraine, fatigue, depression, anxiety, phobias, skin diseases, diarrhoea, asthma and hay fever can occur as a result of the ingestion of certain foods. The most common foods causing reactions are:

- Sugar and sugar-containing foods
- Milk and dairy products
- Chocolate
- Alcoholic beverages
- Tea and coffee
- Wheat
- Other grains and corn
- Shellfish
- Eggs and chicken
- Nuts
- Fish

However, any food can cause a reaction. Frequently, the foods we like a lot, or even crave, are the ones that are causing our symptoms. Food allergy is like an addiction to drugs, although not as severe. Whereas an alcoholic or smoker reach for their glass of beer or cigarette to prevent uncomfortable withdrawal symptoms (tension, pain, shakes, etc.), a good allergy victim may need a sugar or coffee 'fix' to keep them going. Arthritis sufferers frequently enjoy dairy products and foods from the Solanaceae family — tomatoes, potatoes, capsicum and eggplant. The daily consumption of these foods may relieve some symptoms of an allergy, such as fatigue, but simultaneously cause other symptoms such as joint pains and stiffness.

The cardinal sign of a food allergy is one of a 'swinging' constitution. This means that both physical and mental symptoms will swing from one extreme to another. A person may be perfectly normal until exposure to a food allergy and then suddenly or slowly 'swing' into a severe mental depression with no physical energy at all. Or they may develop a mental high followed by a massive migraine. The symptoms of allergy are indicated in the following table:

Common symptoms of food and chemical sensitivities

The nervous system

Fatigue
Sleepiness
Drowsiness
Depression
Spontaneous weepiness and crying
Anxiety
Irritability
Overactivity and overstimulation
Mania and manic attacks
Hyperactivity in children
The hyperactive learning disabled child
Poor short-term memory
Inability to concentrate
Shortened attention span
Misreading words and sentences
Reading without the ability to comprehend
Variations in the ability to read
Stuttering and stammering
Speech disorders
Disturbances in the legibility of hand writing
Tremor, convulsions and fits
Some forms of epilepsy or fits
Restlessness and jitteriness
Irrational fears
Unprovoked aggression
Spontaneous panic attacks
Agitation, tension and aggression
Mental dullness
Mental confusion

Emotional silliness
Symptoms of mental retardation
Claustrophobia
False beliefs (delusions)
Irrational fears (paranoia)
Unexplained inability to move (catatonia)
Paralysis of a temporary nature
Hallucinations (seeing or hearing things that are not there)
Floating sensations in the body and head
A fullness or a pressure in the head
Headaches
Migraines
Personality changes which are cyclical (come and go)

Musculo-skeletal system (muscles and bones)

General muscle weakness
Muscle fatigue
Muscle soreness
Back pain
Chest pains (not caused by heart or lung disease)
Muscle and joint stiffness
Limitation of muscle movement
Spasms in the muscles especially of the hips and shoulders
Generalised muscle pain
Joint pains
Arthritis
Stiffness in the joints
Swelling of joints

Gastro-intestinal system

Heartburn and indigestion
Rumbling in the stomach
Undiagnosed abdominal pains
Colic in infants
Stomach cramps
Alternating diarrhoea and constipation
Undigested food in stools

Flatulence (passing excessive gas)
Mucus in the stool
Colitis (including blood in the bowel action)
'Gall bladder' attacks
Symptoms of stomach or duodenal ulcers
An itchy anus
Burning sensation of the rectum
Nausea and/or vomiting after certain foods
Difficulty in swallowing
Regurgitation and burping
A change in taste sensation
A loss of taste sensation
Metallic taste
Burning or stinging tongue
Geographic tongue (A tongue with unusual patterns on its surface)
Excessive hunger or thirst
Mouth ulcers
Excess dryness of the mouth
Profuse salivation
Irritable bowel syndrome
Pains over the liver
Tenderness of the liver on deep palpation

Skin

Red rashes
Red spots
Very small fine blisters
Large blisters
Hives
Itchiness
Flushing (especially on the face, upper chest and neck areas)
Burning sensations
Increased sensitivity (especially to touch)
Ticklish
Tingling sensations
Peeling of the skin
Pimples
Some forms of acne

Excess sweating
Poor circulation (including Raynaud's syndrome especially affecting fingers and toes)

Ear, nose and throat (ENT)

Runny nose
Sneezing
Nasal itchiness
Post-nasal drip
Nasal stuffiness
Nasal obstruction
Itching ears
Earache deafness — some forms
Dizziness
Vertigo
Disturbances of balance
Ringing in the ears
Persistent undiagnosable 'cough'

Recurrent sore throats
Dry mouth
Itchy or ticklish throat
Red eyes
Swollen eyelids
Itchy eyelids
Twitching eyelids
Watery eyes
Painful eyes
Aching eyes
Eyes tender to touch
Blurring of vision
Double vision
Crossed eyes (sometimes)

The respiratory system

Cough which is undiagnosable
Shortness of breath
Wheezing
Mucus formation
Tightness in the chest
Rapid breathing rate

Cardiovascular system

Blood pressure (some cases)
Palpitations
A pounding heart
Rapid heart rate
Missed or skipped beats

Faintness
Unusual sensations in the chest
Hot flushes
Cold extremities

Tingling of the hands
Extreme redness or blueness of the hands

The genito-urinary system

Increased frequency of urination
Urgency to urinate
Painful urination
Inability to control bladder
A burning sensation
Cloudy urine (exclude infection)
Wetting the bed

Painful genitals
Itching and swelling of the genitals
Vaginal discharge
Penile discharge
Painful intercourse

The above symptoms are not exhaustive of the field of allergy and it must be remembered that some of the symptoms may also occur in serious organic disease, for example 'heartburn and indigestion' may be caused by a peptic ulcer or even coronary artery disease of the heart.

Addictions to any food or chemical can cause the reactions above. In the early stages of the development of an allergy, only one or two symptoms may be present but as time progresses, more problems arise.

Case study

> Elaine Coventry suffered from eczema as a baby, developing asthma that persisted until she was in her mid-seventies. 'I thought that my years of suffering and taking medication had come to an end', said Elaine, now 75 years of age and in radiant good health. 'But my ecstasy was short-lived. After the asthma stopped, I slumped into a deep depression and needed hospitalisation for months.
>
> For the next twenty years I was treated for this severe depression, and I was hospitalised many times. By the age of 50 I had been operated on for gall-bladder and my uterus was removed. After one of the operations, I was violently sick and could not eat for a week. Surprisingly, at the end of this time I had lost the cloud hanging over me, my mind was clear and I was able to laugh again for the first time in many years. This lasted until the third day after I

recommenced eating. I had eaten chicken on that day and within a few minutes I felt nauseated, developed stomach pains like indigestion and my mood suddenly went totally flat. In fact, I could not even think straight. Albert, my husband, suspected that I had suffered from some sort of food poisoning or allergy to chicken and decided to put me on an elimination diet. That was 25 years ago, a time when most people had very little idea of allergy.

Since then I have had only one slight episode of depression after eating a small piece of chicken hidden in a pie.'

This case history clearly illustrates the change in nature of allergy symptoms over time from eczema, asthma, depression, gallbladder pain and possibly even gynaecological disorders (heavy painful periods requiring hysterectomy). Unfortunately, Elaine Coventry was allergic to the smallest amount of chicken. Sometimes allergies are not as severe and small quantities of the offending substance are safe.

Stress reduces the tolerance to allergenic foods. On holidays, Steven Wright could drink milk and eat oranges, but back at work he developed itchy skin rashes and migraines when these foods were consumed.

The allergic/addicted person usually has multiple symptoms and multiple offending foods. The problems usually start in early childhood with an allergy to something like dairy products. If the dairy products cause common symptoms including fatigue, tiredness and irritability, it isn't long before the young person starts looking for sugar for a quick energy 'pick-me-up'. Eventually the effect of the sugar wears off and to achieve a 'high' or an altered state, alcohol, tobacco or even cocaine or marijuana are tried. Most allergy/addicted people of retirement age are caught up with coffee, tea, sugar, alcohol and/or tobacco - the 'harder' substances being made readily available only in later years to the youth of the 60s, 70s and 80s.

Most allergy sufferers of retirement age today have problems with common foods (and sometimes chemicals), and as the incriminated foods are often 'hidden' in the diet, the allergies may be masked. This makes the diagnosis somewhat difficult.

How does one determine what food or chemical is causing or aggravating symptoms?

Various tests can be performed. Fasting, the avoidance of all food for 3-4 days, following by provocation with food challenges and the recording of symptoms, is time consuming and difficult. Sublingual tests in which dilute suspensions of a large series of foods are placed under the tongue one by one to elicit allergic reactions are also time consuming. Skin tests and prick tests are inaccurate. The pulse test involves the measurement of the pulse rate at the wrist before and after eating a single food. If the pulse rate changes by more than plus or minus 16 beats a minute, then an allergic reaction to that food may have occurred.

Electronic tests such as the Theratest and Vegatest are useful guides, quick and inexpensive. Their scientific validation has yet to be proven but many thousands of people have benefitted from them.

One of the most accurate methods of testing is to measure the amount of special antibody (IgE and IgG4 antibody) to various foods. This test is very specific and is a measure of 'true allergy'. Used in conjunction with elimination of suspected foods and 'stress' foods, most allergy sufferers can achieve very satisfactory results.

Elimination of stress foods means total avoidance of sugar, white flour, alcohol, tea, coffee, chocolate, all dairy foods, tobacco, yeast-containing foods and chemical additives. Always suspect foods eaten regularly and foods that are 'liked' or 'disliked'. Often the food that is most resistant to elimination from the diet because of desire is the food most likely to cause the problem.

It is important to remember that if a food that causes allergy has been removed from the diet for more than a week and the symptoms have completely cleared up, the reintroduction of the offending food may result in severe, dramatic allergic reactions such as vomiting, headaches, stomach cramps, wheezing, lethargy, tiredness and so on.

This brings me to the most effective way to treat all of these allergy reactions. The most logical and commonsense thing to do is to avoid the causative foods and chemicals. If this is not possible completely because of lifestyle, or the diagnosis of all allergies proves difficult, then the use of supportive nutrients for the immune system, nervous system and any other affected systems is imperative.

One of the most useful nutrients is vitamin C with bioflavonoids in oral doses of 2 to 4 grams per day. If allergies are very severe, many doctors around the world will give intravenous injections of vitamin C in doses up to 30 grams per day.

Most of the B-complex vitamins help to control many of the symptoms of allergy especially fatigue, lethargy, depression, irritability, fluid retention, poor memory and concentration. These are given in doses of 100-200mgm daily and again can be very effective by injection especially vitamins B12 and folic acid.

The minerals zinc and selenium are extremely important for the proper functioning of the immune system and most allergic people have low levels of these minerals. The recommended dose of elemental zinc is 15 to 30mg per day and the dose of elemental selenium is 200microgram per day. Natural vitamin E in capsule form 250i.u. per day also helps by reducing the oxidising damage often caused by chemical allergies.

The essential fatty acids present in evening primrose oil have been shown to be useful in the allergic patient, especially for the treatment of eczema and arthritis. Six to eight capsules per day are needed to achieve a good result.

There are many good herbal remedies on the market that can be used to alleviate the annoying symptoms of allergy, some herbs may even have the ability to nourish affected tissues back to health.

Homeopathic medicines properly prescribed are also very safe and effective.

Allergy injections cannot be recommended for most allergies and may actually aggravate the condition.

A final and very important part of the management is fresh air, sunlight, exercise and a positive outlook. Exercises most beneficial are swimming, walking, cycling and yoga or tai chi. Scientists have proven that exercise increases the bodies ability to produce certain 'well-being' chemicals including the pain-relieving endorphins and immune system regulators. With regular exercise, the right foods and the judicious use of vitamins and minerals, life can be an allergy-free and disease-free joy for all.

Food chemical sensitivity and fatigue

One of the most common causes of fatigue and tiredness is a sensitivity to foods or chemicals, including drugs and medications.

Chemicals present as pollutants in our foods, water and air can act as very potent fatigue-inducers in many people. In fact, quite often the only symptom of such a sensitivity in the early stages of an illness is the symptom of fatigue.

In patients with food and chemical sensitivities, single and multiple nutritional deficiency states are often observed. This is usually of the water soluble nutrients such as the B-group vitamins and vitamin C. These appear to be utilised quite rapidly when the body is under extra physical or psychological stress.

It is unsatisfactory for a person suffering with fatigue and allergies to have a simple blood test to determine the adequacy of their nutritional status. Quite often it is essential to perform highly specific tests in special laboratories before a nutritional deficiency or imbalance state can be diagnosed. For example, a deficiency of the element zinc can result in mental apathy, tiredness, poor memory, mood changes and acne. Tests to determine the amount of zinc in the blood, even in patients with a clinical deficiency, may be normal. Sometimes it is more appropriate to look inside the cells of the body and tissues to determine more accurately the body's zinc status. Zinc is associated with enzyme function and many enzymes are dependent upon an adequate supply of zinc. Therefore another test for zinc adequacy is the measurement of the activity of enzymes in the patient. Another test is the zinc tolerance test in which zinc levels in the blood and urine are measured before and after the individual swallows a measured amount of zinc. The zinc taste test in which the patient is given a solution of zinc salts is a moderately accurate method of assessing zinc status. A 0.9% solution of zinc sulphate in water is given to the person being tested and if there is no taste or a dry and furry sensation to the solution, then a zinc deficiency is likely. Adequate zinc status is suggested by an immediate taste which may be metallic, strong and quite unpleasant.

Here we see many tests that can be performed for the

assessment of just one single nutrient. These tests are not done routinely in normal pathology laboratories. It is therefore very important to investigate which is the most appropriate test for the particular situation.

Food and chemical sensitivities

The brain and nervous system are extremely complex chemical factories. Their function depends totally on the supply of blood containing essential nutrients including oxygen and water, and the removal of wastes through the bloodstream. The essential nutrients are oxygen, glucose, water, amino acids from protein, essential fatty acids, vitamins, minerals and trace elements. These nutrients for the brain are derived from our diet. Many of these nutrients act as building blocks for the maintenance of brain cells and nervous tissue. Others are important as chemical messengers, also known as neurotransmitters. These chemical messengers travel from one brain cell to another carrying with them information to keep the nervous system functioning properly. The majority of these chemical messengers (neurotransmitters) are derived from protein in our diet and are known as amino acids. Some examples of these amino acids which become neurotransmitters are tryptophan, tyrosine, lysine, glutamine and phenylalanine.

The production and metabolism of many of these neurotransmitters and building blocks for the nervous system are dependent on adequate supplies of bulk minerals, trace elements and vitamins to the nervous system as well. The most important of these nutrients are vitamins C, B1, B2, B3, B6, B12, folic acid, zinc, calcium and magnesium. If the diet is unbalanced or low in any of these nutrients then the first systems to suffer usually are the central nervous system and the immune system. As a consequence, the functioning of the brain and nervous system alters and this is reflected in a wide diversity of symptoms including fatigue, lethargy, insomnia, dizziness, visual disturbances, loss of co-ordination, muscle weakness, nervousness, anxiety, tension, depression and even such symptoms as paranoia, delusional thinking, loss of ability to concentrate and poor short-term memory. In severe cases, gross deficiencies of some of these nutrients can result in delirium, coma, fitting and even death.

It is important to remember that any organ or tissue in the body can react in an allergic or sensitive manner to foods and chemicals in the environment. This is particularly so in the case of the brain and nervous system. It was stated hundreds of years ago that what is one man's food is another man's poison and what one individual can tolerate in the way of a food, another may react to in a very sensitive manner.

Food and chemical allergies or sensitivities are not only responsible for classical allergies such as asthma, hay fever and eczema, but they can also be responsible for other physical allergies such as the irritable bowel syndrome, bowel disease in general, skin rashes, acne, dermatitis and migraine headaches.

Generally, food and chemical sensitivities can aggravate nearly every known disease.

CHAPTER SEVEN

Malnutrition in chronic fatigue syndrome

Lucy's story

Running her own health store and working as a therapeutic masseuse at night became too much for Lucy, a 26 year old vegetarian. She had seen a number of doctors, psychologists and even a psychiatrist to try to sort out why she was so irritable, tired and depressed and unable to function the way she had in the past.

She had no obvious signs of any serious medical illness and no relevant past history except that her mother suffered from pernicious anaemia in her early 40s. Pernicious anaemia is a killer disease which occurs as a consequence of the body's inability to absorb adequate amounts of vitamin B12 from the diet. It is treated by the monthly injection of 1000mg of vitamin B12. Many medical scientists now believe that pernicious anaemia is an expression of a malfunctioning immune and gastrointestinal system with a tendency for these malfunctions to run in families. Lucy's blood tests showed a vitamin B12 level at the lower level of normal. She was not actually deficient in vitamin B12, but the low level was probably responsible for her fatigue, anxiety and depression. Shortly after Lucy's first injection of vitamin B12 her energy levels zapped up dramatically to what they had been. She required an injection of B12 weekly to maintain her energy levels.

It was also discovered that dried apricots were another cause of Lucy's fatigue. Experimentation and elimination of apricot products revealed that Lucy was not allergic to apricots but to the sulphite preservatives used in the drying process. It is interesting to note here that the enzymes required to detoxify the body of sulphites are vitamin B12 dependent. Lucy's fatigue improved even further when sulphites were eliminated, as much as possible, from her environment and diet.

Lucy continued to require vitamin B12 injections every month to six weeks to maintain a level of wellness conducive to her active lifestyle.

How many times have you heard it said that if you eat a well-balanced standard diet you will obtain all of the nutrients necessary for good health? Until recently, most doctors and dieticians sincerely believed that this was the truth.

However, hard scientific evidence has recently shown that over 150 different medical conditions are associated with multiple nutritional deficiency states. Many of these conditions are directly or indirectly the result of poor diet and have been shown to be responsive to a change in diet and nutritional supplementation. The following list clearly illustrates those who are at risk of malnutrition.

Population sub-groups at risk of malnutrition

1. Adolescents
2. Alcoholics
3. People who consume more than two alcoholic drinks per day
4. Smokers and drug users
5. Vegetarians (some)

6. Low socio-economic groups
7. The obese
8. People on weight reducing programs
9. The aged and infirm
10. People on medication
11. People on fad diets
12. People on high fibre diets
13. Aborigines
14. Pregnant women
15. The busy professional or executive eating on the run
16. Patients receiving intravenous nutrition

From this list it can be seen that probably only a very small percentage of Australians do not fit into any of the categories and that many Australians would satisfy two or even three.

What relevance does this have to the patient with the chronic fatigue syndrome? It has been documented that single or multiple nutritional deficiencies of such nutrients as vitamins, trace elements, minerals, essential fatty acids, amino acids, protein, or carbohydrates can cause a wide range of symptoms including fatigue. In fact, an interesting study on thiamine (vitamin B1) has shown that the concentration of thiamine in the blood of patients with fatigue and tiredness may be normal yet the use of 100mg to 200mg (megadose) of thiamine daily in these patients will eliminate the fatigue and associated symptoms in the majority of this group. This point illustrates the necessity to de-emphasise the value of blood tests in the clinical situation.

Another example is vitamin B6 (pyridoxine) in asthmatic patients. It appears that there is an abnormality in the way that asthmatic patients handle vitamin B6. A number of studies have shown that asthmatic patients can benefit dramatically from the use of high dose B6. In fact it requires high maintenance doses of B6 to achieve a satisfactory blood level of this particular vitamin in asthmatics. As a consequence of this and other nutritional manoeuvres, asthmatics can reduce their requirements for cortisone and broncodilator drugs and even dramatically cut their hospital admission rate.

This brings us again to the point of biochemical individuality. We all have different requirements for various nutrients and in some disease states, to achieve the optimum state of nutrition and therefore health, supplementary doses are necessary. The following table illustrates those nutrients which, if low in the diet or interfered with by drugs, chemicals, heavy metals or medication may result in easy fatiguing.

Nutrient inadequacies associated with fatigue

The nutrients below, if not provided in optimum concentrations in the diet, or if needed in greater quantities than are obtainable in the diet at times of increased stress, have all been shown scientifically to result in fatigue (and many other symptoms).

Biotin	Pantothenic acid (vitamin B5)
Calcium	Para-aminobenzoic acid (PABA)
Chromium	Phosphorus
Copper	Potassium
Essential fatty acids, e.g. from fish oil and evening primrose oil	Pyridoxine (vitamin B6)
	Riboflavin
	Sodium
Folic acid	Thiamine (vitamin B1)
Inadequate carbohydrate intake	Vitamin A
Protein malnutrition	Vitamin B12 (best administered by intramuscular injection)
Iodine	
Iron	Vitamin C (fatigue is an early sign of vitamin C malnourishment)
Magnesium	
Manganese	
Niacin (vitamin B3)	Zinc

It is not necessary to have an absolute deficiency of any single nutrient before the early signs and symptoms of a deficiency appear. For example, low levels of folic acid can result in poor memory, apathy, irritability and fatigue — all of which can be corrected by supplementing the diet.

Blood tests on patients with these symptoms usually show a blood level of folic acid in the low-normal range of values. Many doctors therefore conclude that the test result is within the normal range and can be ignored. However, this is not necessarily the case and low-normal blood tests may actually reflect a deficiency state in the deeper tissues, for example, the muscle cells, red blood cells, brain cells etc.

Another factor affecting the efficiency of vitamins and nutrients is the presence of an inhibiting substance, for example a xenobiotic chemical or heavy metal. An example of this is the effect of lead on the antioxidant capabilities of the red blood cells and its effect in increasing the requirements for vitamin B1. Sulphites present in preserved meats, dried fruits, polluted air and wine can interfere with the metabolic activity of vitamin B12 thus increasing the requirements for vitamin B12 in sulphite sensitive individuals.

In patients with the chronic fatigue syndrome it has been found that over 80% of patients have increased requirements for low levels of vitamin C, over 70% of patients have increased requirements for, or low levels of, at least one of the B-complex vitamins and that chromium, zinc and selenium are the minerals most often found to be deficient in the low normal range. The following tables illustrate the signs and symptoms of nutritional inadequacies in the CFS patient. An examination of these deficiency signs and symptoms is highly recommended for the sufferer of the chronic fatigue syndrome.

Remember, blood tests are notoriously inaccurate in the assessment of the tissue status of these nutrients, especially if the level is borderline or low-normal on the blood test.

Signs and symptoms of vitamin C deficiency (before scurvy occurs)

1. Lassitude and fatigue
2. Listlessness
3. Confusion
4. Depression
5. Breathlessness
6. Sallow complexion
7. Disinterest in exercise or activity
8. Loss of appetite
9. A mild anaemia
10. Desire for increased sleep
11. Fleeting pains in the joints

12. Easy bruising
13. Scurvy then develops in which gums bleed, teeth fall out, severe weakness, pneumonia or death occurs.

Signs and symptoms of vitamin B1 deficiency (thiamine)

1. Fatigue and tiredness
2. Apathy
3. Emotional instability
4. Depression
5. Confusion of thought
6. Feeling of impending doom
7. Abdominal symptoms and indigestion
8. Diarrhoea and constipation
9. Anorexia and weight loss
10. Low pain tolerance
11. Anaemia
12. Shortness of breath
13. Numbness in the hands or feet
14. A burning sensation in the hands or feet
15. Increased sensitivity to noise
16. Palpitations of the heart
17. A slowing of metabolic rate (feeling cold)
18. In severe cases, heart failure occurs

Signs and symptoms of vitamin B2 deficiency (riboflavin)

1. Cracks in the corners of the mouth
2. Cracks in the lips
3. Insomnia
4. Slowing of mental processes
5. Oily scaly skin
6. Hair loss
7. Dizziness and trembling
8. A red, sometimes painful tongue
9. Cataract formation in the eyes

Signs and symptoms of a vitamin B3 deficiency (niacin)

1. Depression, fatigue and a sense of gloom and doom
2. Fears, phobias and suspicion
3. Worry and apprehension
4. Changes in behaviour including antisocial behaviour
5. Muscle weakness
6. Insomnia
7. Burning sensations
8. Disturbances in perception (schizophrenia type symptoms)
9. A red tipped tongue
10. Dental indentations at the margins of the tongue
11. Swollen, painful and sometimes bleeding gums
12. Sore mouth
13. Halitosis (bad breath)
14. Irritable bowel symptoms and indigestion
15. Excessive flatulence
16. Poorly formed, offensive stools
17. Undiagnosable abdominal pain
18. Dermatitis
19. Allergies and chemical sensitivities
20. Dementia and death occur from pellagra if severe.

Signs and symptoms of vitamin B5 deficiency (pantothenic acid)

1. Fatigue
2. Depression
3. Insomnia
4. Pains in the middle of the back (over the adrenal glands)
5. Frequent infections
6. Anorexia
7. Constipation
8. Burning feet syndrome

Signs and symptoms of vitamin B6 deficiency (pyridoxine)

1. Many nervous symptoms including tension and anxiety
2. Depression
3. Iron resistant anaemia
4. Epileptic type fits
5. Fluid retention and swelling
6. Oily scales on the scalp, nose and eyebrows
7. Dandruff
8. Numbness in the hands
9. Cramping in the arms and legs
10. Cracking on the mouth and hands
11. Nausea
12. Morning sickness (in pregnancy)
13. Some forms of arthritis or arthralgia
14. Some symptoms of the premenstrual syndrome
15. Pallor of the skin without anaemia

Signs and symptoms of folic acid deficiency

1. Apathy and lethargy
2. Irritability
3. Slowing of intellectual functions
4. Total withdrawal and isolation
5. Poor short-term memory
6. Cracks in the corners of the mouth
7. Malabsorption of nutrients
8. Megaloblastic Anaemia
9. Muscle weakness
10. Paranoid ideation

Signs and symptoms of vitamin B12 deficiency

1. Apathy
2. Fatigue
3. Poor short-term memory
4. Deficiency in concentration

5. Mood swings
6. Learning disorders
7. Confusion
8. Hallucinations in some
9. Paranoia and irrational fears
10. A red shiny smooth tongue
11. Severe tiredness and nervousness
12. If severe, pernicious anaemia and degeneration of the spinal cord
13. Senility

Signs and symptoms of a biotin deficiency

1. Fatigue
2. Depression
3. Anorexia
4. Nausea
5. Hair Loss
6. High cholesterol levels
7. High blood sugar levels (like diabetes)
8. Muscle weakness, muscle pains
9. Insomnia
10. Dry skin
11. Greyish pallor
12. Increased sensitivity to touch
13. Drowsiness
14. Dermatitis without itch
15. Abnormal electrocardiogram

Signs and symptoms of zinc deficiency (common in the chronic fatigue syndrome)

1. Fatigue
2. Loss of taste sensation
3. Irritability
4. Lethargy
5. Depression
6. Apathy
7. Anorexia and loss of appetite
8. Deterioration of short-term memory
9. Eczema
10. Brittle nails
11. Delayed sexual maturity and impotence in males
12. Gross impairment
13. Hair loss
14. Acne
15. Impaired wound healing
16. Impairment of short-term memory

17. Irrational fears
18. White spots on the fingernails
19. Sterility
20. Abnormal blood sugar control (hypoglycaemia and diabetes)
21. Stretch marks on the skin
22. Irregular menstrual periods
23. Painful joints and arthritis
24. Frequent upper respiratory tract infections
25. Enlargement of the prostrate
26. Severe emotional and behaviourial disorders
27. Susceptibility to chemical sensitivity

Signs and symptoms of chromium deficiency

1. Fatigue and tiredness
2. Anxiety
3. Impairment of growth
4. Glucose intolerance (swinging blood sugar eventually resulting in diabetes)
5. High blood cholesterol
6. Possible joint pains
7. Sugar and refined carbohydrate cravings (including alcohol and white flour products)

Signs and symptoms of selenium deficiency

1. Frequent infections (including viral infections)
2. Sterility in males
3. Impairment of liver function
4. High blood cholesterol
5. Inflammation in the skin or gastrointestinal tract
6. Heightened sensitivity to chemicals (chemical hyper-sensitivity/allergy)

Signs and symptoms of essential fatty acid deficiency

1. Dry skin
2. Dry brittle hair
3. Eczema
4. Diarrhoea
5. Hair loss
6. Impairment of growth
7. Disturbances in hormone functioning
8. Acne
9. Disturbances in liver function
10. Gallstone formation
11. Impairment of growth
12. Disturbances in function of the immune system
13. Impairment of wound healing
14. Kidney disorders
15. Infertility
16. Mental symptoms of anxiety, depression and irritability
17. Poor nail growth
18. Arthralgia and joint pains
19. Muscle weakness

The importance of antioxidants

In Chapter 5 — *Chemicals, Drugs and Free Radical Disease* the role of antioxidants was discussed and their ability to mop up damaging free radicals was emphasised. The increasing hard scientific evidence supports the unifying hypothesis that the chronic fatigue syndrome is a dysfunction of multi-systems precipitated by a combination of factors conferring an excessive and inappropriate oxidative damage by free radicals.

Of all of the antioxidants discussed in Chapter 5 the easiest to measure and evaluate are the non-enzymatic antioxidants. The non-enzymatic antioxidants are ascorbic acid (vitamin C), reduced glutathione, vitamin E, beta-carotene, uric acid and the copper containing protein caeruloplasmin. Zinc, manganese and selenium levels are also useful. Of these antioxidants, ascorbic acid is uniformly low in the majority of patients. Zinc and selenium are also generally low and in approximately 25% of patients selenium may be regarded as being deficient.

The prime free radical scavenger in the water soluble compartments of the body is vitamin C. Vitamin C and its deficiency state — scurvy — have influenced the course of history. Scurvy was known to the ancient Egyptians and to the great explorers of the world — Jacques Cartier, Sir Richard Hawkins and Captain James Cook, who was the first to successfully use fresh fruit to prevent this disease taking its toll on sailors during prolonged sea voyages.

Even after the discovery by James Lind in 1747 on the H.M.S. **Salisbury** that fresh lemons and limes reverse the symptoms of scurvy, it took the British Admiralty a number of decades before this practice was adopted in the Royal Navy. It was estimated that after fresh fruit was supplied to sailors the effective fighting force of the British Fleet was increased by a factor of 300%. However, it appears that we must repeat our mistakes to continue learning. For example, Scott's death in Antarctica in 1912 was due to scurvy and rampant scurvy persisted throughout the American Civil War.

In modern societies we don't see overt scurvy, but in clinical practice we constantly see patients with the early signs of vitamin C inadequacy. In real life the development of the full blown deficiency disease scurvy occurs over a number of weeks and results in severe bleeding, possibly pneumonia and death from shock. However, before that develops the early symptoms and signs of low vitamin C activity include lethargy, fatigue, muscle weakness, aches and pains in the joints, tender muscles, sallow skin colour, listlessness, lassitude, confusion and depression.

We don't expect to see deficiency states in our society but they do still occur. The big problem people in most western industrialised nations face is the development of low grade inadequacy states which, over a period of time, result in increased requirements for nutrients above that which is supplied in the daily diet. Many of the symptoms alluded to earlier will respond after simple supplementation with vitamin C. However, if the symptoms are allowed to persist and the vitamin C levels are not increased then stress occurs on other biochemical systems resulting in an increased utilisation of other B-complex vitamins, minerals and nutrients.

Vitamin C should be regarded as the key and principal nutrient in the management of the patient with the chronic fatigue syndrome. To explain this we must first understand what the actions of vitamin C are in the body. Firstly, it is a very powerful reducing agent (antioxidant) and free radical scavenger. It stimulates the immune system by increasing the white cell's ability to engulf bacteria and viruses and kill them, it improves the functions of the helper cells and natural killer cells, and it improves the production of interferon and other immune chemicals.

Vitamin C has been shown to inhibit the replication of viruses and the reproduction of bacteria. It modifies the production of prostaglandins, and it has a natural antihistaminic, anti-allergy action. Some studies have even shown vitamin C to inhibit the formation of cancer cells and it has been shown to suppress leukaemic cells and melanoma. Vitamin C may prevent dysplasia of the female cervix, and it is also anti-carcinogenic with respect to cancer of the bladder. The formation of nitrosamines and other carcinogens in the gut is also prevented by the action of vitamin C. Cyclic AMP, an important compound involved in the metabolic processes of most body cells, is also stimulated by ascorbic acid. Vitamin C improves the function, and stimulates the activity, of liver enzymes, especially those involved in the processes of chemical detoxification.

Finally, some studies have shown that vitamin C actually improves the effects of radiotherapy and chemotherapy in cancer.

Eric's cancer

> 'It's a miracle,' said 70 year old Eric as he climbed off the couch. 'I didn't realise that I could feel so well again. I had resolved that my numbered days would be miserable.' Eric had been diagnosed with inoperable cancer of the large bowel. He had secondary cancer in the liver and glands of the abdomen and the cancer had spread locally to attach itself to other organs in the pelvis.
>
> He had been told by his cancer specialist that he would live for between two weeks and two months and that an impending bowel obstruction from the cancerous mass would necessitate hospitalisation and palliative surgery. Eric's bowel actions were loose, fluid and associated with much gas, pain and abdominal bloating. He was understandably

frightened. Back pain, possibly from invasion of nerves in the back by cancer cells, was being controlled with massage and gentle manipulation by his chiropractor. The chiropractor, having been trained in nutrition and continuing with an interest in the field of therapeutic nutrition, had heard of the work of Linus Pauling and Lady Phyllis Cilento using vitamin C for patients with cancer. Eric was advised to start taking vitamin C in megadoses by mouth and to find a doctor who would administer intravenous megavitamin C regularly.

Eric commenced intravenous vitamin C at very low doses to start with — 7.5-15g — and decided to have the injections daily. After the first day he did not notice any change in his condition and continued on to the second, third, fourth and fifth days without any noticeable change. However, at the end of a week he noticed that his bowels were not as loose and that some formed motion was being passed. He also noticed that there was less pain and bloating in the abdomen and that it continued to improve over the next four weeks.

At the end of six weeks of treatment Eric made the wonderful discovery that during his intravenous ascorbate programme his activity levels had gradually but significantly increased. In fact, the severe fatigue he had learned to live with over the past two years prior to diagnosis of cancer had miraculously disappeared. He still suffered from intermittent bouts of fatigue but the debilitating, depressing and demoralizing tiredness — his cancer syndrome — had gone. In fact, Eric improved his diet, took appropriate nutrient supplements and continued intravenous vitamin C for over two years after his initial prognosis of two months had lapsed.

This particular case history illustrates how sometimes the use of one single nutrient and virtually little else can help a patient with chronic fatigue. However, it is not usually as simple as this case illustrates and many factors must be taken into consideration when determining the treatment of any individual patient. Most importantly, in all the investigation of a patient with chronic and severe fatigue, all other possible treatable organic causes of fatigue must be eliminated. These include diseases of the heart and lungs, underlying lymphoma, leukaemia, cancer, diabetes, auto-immune diseases, anaemia, depression, functional reactive hypoglycaemia, the organic brain syndrome (drug and chemical toxicity), chronic dental infection and low thyroid function. Only then can one start to evaluate the nutritional and environmental factors that play a role in most of the fatigue syndromes encountered in the community.

Much more research needs to be done in these areas but this very brief discussion of its actions has top scientists around the world excited about the potential for vitamin C and its co-antioxidants in both the prevention and treatment of disease into the 21st century.

We have investigated the role of infectious micro-organisms in the possible causation of the chronic fatigue syndrome. A thorough search of the scientific and medical literature reveals that vitamin C has been investigated in thousands of studies of infectious disease and it has been shown to have an adverse effect on a wide range of micro-organisms. The diseases studied include herpes simplex (cold sores and genital herpes), infectious hepatitis, glandular fever, german measles, the common cold, influenza and bacterial infections including pseudomonas, urinary tract infections and rabies (in guinea pigs). The outcome of an infectious disease is determined by the state of health of the individual at the time of the infection. In particular, the nutritional health of the patient at the time of initial infection determines to a large degree the course of that infection. With acute viral infections such as glandular fever, hepatitis, influenza and the common cold, the use of vitamin C as an antioxidant and antimicrobial agent by intravenous infusion has gained worldwide favour. Its most effective use is at the first sign or symptom of an infection occurring. Doses of between 15gm and 60gm may be necessary. Dramatic clinical responses can be obtained with these and other infections including viral meningitis and chicken pox in adults.

Nicki's chicken pox and glandular fever

> Nicki, aged 18, suffered from adult chicken pox that severely affected her mouth, gullet and airways. Chicken pox in an

adult can be so severe that it may result in fatal pneumonia. Nicki was seen by her doctor late in the night at her home after having seen a GP earlier in the day who prescribed antibiotics. She was extremely ill and the pain in her throat was so severe that she couldn't even swallow her own saliva.

The ideal treatment in a case like this is hospitalisation and intravenous fluids. Intravenous megadose vitamin C usually aborts the infection very quickly without the necessity for hospitalisation but unfortunately her doctor didn't have the necessary supply in his emergency bag. However, he did give her an injection of megadose vitamins B1, B6, B12 and folic acid and to their amazement her pain disappeared in minutes and she was able to take fluids orally. Nicki's throat, which had been inflamed and full of chicken pox blisters, was looking much healthier two hours after the injection.

This rapid response to a megadose vitamin B intramuscular injection should have alerted the doctor to the possibility that Nicki may have suffered from a vitamin deficiency or dependency state which predisposed her to such a severe attack. Unfortunately, it didn't and although Nicki rapidly recovered from this infection she developed glandular fever four months later while overseas and was given no active treatment at all. She arrived back home totally exhausted and couldn't work for months. It wasn't until she saw her 'vitamin doctor' that she realised how effective the vitamin treatment had been for her chicken pox. After four injections of the high potency B-complex (as described in Chapter 10 on the treatment of CFS), Nicki regained her usual strength and energy with the enthusiasm for her filmmaking that had originally taken her overseas.

In considering other major factors contributing to the chronic fatigue syndrome — that is, the heavy metals, mercury and lead and the possible contributing role that synthetic chemicals play — the other major activity of vitamin C as a potent detoxifying agent cannot be over-emphasised. Vitamin C detoxifies against the harmful effects of such chemicals as strychnine, digitalis poisoning (a heart drug), sulphur drugs, vitamin A toxicity, alcohol, barbiturates, morphine, anaesthetics, many medical drugs, benzene and other synthetics and it has an antagonistic effect on lead, mercury, arsenic, carbon dioxide, sulphur dioxide and cancer drugs. It has detoxifying effects on diphtheria toxin, tetanus toxin, botulism and even snake and spider bites. This marvellous molecule has the potential for playing a major role in most human diseases and treatments.

In patients with the chronic fatigue syndrome, courses of intravenous vitamin C are invaluable. Daily injections between 15gm and 60gm intravenously are recommended. The form of vitamin C is sodium ascorbate. It is extremely safe given intravenously over a period of 15 to 20 minutes. The only major side effect is a sclerosing of the vein and pain over the injection site if the ascorbate happens to leak out of the vein.

One of the greatest medical myths ever created is that of the damaging effect of vitamin C on the kidneys. There is no good evidence to support the theory that vitamin C causes kidney damage and, in fact, vitamin C is used in the treatment and prevention of some kidney disorders. If megadoses of vitamin C were so harmful to the kidney by producing kidney stones we would be witnessing an epidemic throughout the western world, because of the massive doses that large sections of the population have been taking over the last fifteen to twenty years. This is not the case. Also, rebound scurvy, that is vitamin C deficiency on sudden withdrawal of large doses, does not occur.

The destruction of vitamin B12 by vitamin C is another fallacy based on faulty laboratory techniques. Vitamin C is safe to use provided it is used in the manner outlined in Chapter 10. For the chronic fatigue syndrome patient, daily injections may need to be continued for two to three weeks combined with a general nutrition and supplementation programme which may need to be extended for six to twelve months.

Chronic fatigue syndrome patients who have responded to treatment in the past and who develop more viral infections after regaining their health should immediately recommence the intravenous vitamin C. In this way the viral infection can be aborted and the risk of the re-development of fatigue is minimised.

In severe cases, the use of vitamin C alone is futile. In nutrition, teamwork is essential. Every nutrient is like a different instrument in an orchestra and each nutrient plays a part in the nutritional symphony. Just as the antioxidants interact with one another, so do most of the other nutrients. For example, if vitamin C is going to stimulate immune function, it cannot do so if the patient is deficient in zinc or the B-complex vitamins and/or protein. These other nutrients must be supplied in optimum quantities for the ascorbate to work. It is pointless putting brand new spark plugs into a coked-up old motor car engine that needs new bearings and is running on low grade fuel. It simply will not deliver the performance. As an agent to stimulate the detoxification mechanisms vitamin C requires the help of certain amino acids, for example, the sulphur containing amino acids, methionine and cysteine. These sulphur containing amino acids have groups called sulphydryl groups which combine with the activity of ascorbate and help to detoxify mercury. Taurine is formed from the sulphur containing amino acid cysteine and it is important in the inactivation of the hypochlorite radical, formed from the chlorinated hydrocarbons in chemical pesticides. Cysteine is also important for the production of glutathione, and glutathione is necessary for the activity of glutathione peroxidase antioxidant enzyme.

Vitamin C has been shown to have many other actions as well as those mentioned above. Amongst these is an increased pain threshold and an increase in well-being by having an antidepressant effect on the central nervous system. Although in severe depression ascorbate alone will have only an insignificant effect, in most of the mild to moderate depressions seen in the chronic fatigue syndrome, the constant use of ascorbate orally and by injection is recommended.

Given that vitamin C in the doses recommended here are safe, one must ask the question, 'What are the safety levels of the other nutrients recommended'. Cases of alleged, harmful side effects and adverse reactions to vitamins are occasionally reported in the medical literature and the general press. The support of these allegations is usually anecdotal. Unfortunately, testimonials to the adverse reactions nutritional substances are reiterated by well intentioned or biased writers without any adequate scientific supporting evidence, thus increasing the implied credibility.

In general, it can be said that the levels of vitamins normally ingested by the majority of the population in their diet and in multi-vitamin preparations are very safe. A growing and substantial portion of the nation consume vitamins and minerals at levels in excess of the advised dosages. This practice has been increasing over the past ten years without any evidence of toxicity or harmful side effects. In fact, some research shows that individuals supplementing their diet are in better health than prior to supplementation and are probably at much less risk of developing certain degenerative diseases including cardiovascular disease, diabetes and perhaps even cancer.

There is a very considerable margin of safety with most nutrients including vitamins, minerals and herbs. Compared with drugs, there are very few side effects that can be attributed to vitamins, even at dose levels substantially greater than the recommended daily allowances. In fact, it has been estimated that nutritional supplements are between 1,000 and 10,000 safer than medically prescribed drugs and over-the-counter medications.

Over 20% of some hospital beds are occupied by patients suffering from iatrogenic disease (physician induced drug side effects). The admission to hospital of patients suffering from an overdose of a nutritional supplement is almost unheard of and would consist of only a handful of patients in this country. In fact, there is no documented case of a patient being rushed to hospital in an ambulance from a life-threatening overdose of a vitamin.

The water soluble vitamins, that is the B-complex and C, have an extremely wide margin of safety. Doses in excess of 100 times the recommended daily allowance for the B-complex and 1,000 times the recommended daily allowance for vitamin C have been tolerated well in special groups of patients. However, the recommended maximum doses for all nutrients are given in Chapter 10 and they should not be exceeded. With the exception of the adverse reactions that occur after long-term ingestion of vitamins A, D and B6, vitamin side effects that occur are rapidly reversible on withdrawal of the supplementation. They generally leave minimal and usually no long lasting effects. The message is that nutritional therapy including vitamin supplementation is extremely safe and very effective.

A few words here about the possible side effects of vitamins A, D and B6. An overdose of vitamin A can cause irritability, depression, aches and pains, dry skin, cracking of the lips, hair loss, a yellowing of the skin, headaches, painful eyes and, if severe, enlargement of the liver and raised pressure inside the skull. This only occurs if the overdose of vitamin A is severe. Recommended levels of intakes of vitamin A are approximately 5,000i.u. per day. A safe supplementary dose is 9,000i.u. per day but in some therapeutic situations it may increase to 100,000i.u. per day for short periods under medical supervision. Studies have shown that a safe therapeutic dose of vitamin A is 30,000i.u. per day to 50,000i.u. per day. However, in the chronic fatigue syndrome it is not necessary to dose at this high level. A maximum of 20,000i.u. to 25,000i.u. of vitamin A per day is adequate to maintain a blood level in the upper range.

Excessive vitamin D causes nausea, vomiting, diarrhoea, muscle weakness, fatigue, dizziness and frequency of urination but most importantly it causes deposits of calcium to occur in the soft tissues of the body including the kidneys, heart, blood vessels and around various joints. The recommended intake of vitamin D varies from country to country from 200i.u. to 400i.u. per day. The maximum safe dose has not been determined. This of course is the vitamin that is synthesised in the skin when exposed to sunlight. Reports of toxicity occurring at 25,000i.u. per day have occurred. However, to be safe with this hormone-like vitamin, no more than 1,000i.u. per day can ever be recommended.

The last and probably the most controversial of the toxic vitamins is pyridoxine (vitamin B6). For many years women were using vitamin B6 safely in high doses to treat the symptoms of the premenstrual syndrome. Doses of 100mgs per day, (that is over 50 times the RDA) for periods of up to four years revealed no adverse effects from this nutrient. In fact, some studies indicated that 200mgs per day were safe. Human nature being what it is, some patients decided to medicate in excessive doses of between 4,000 and 6,000mgs per day which resulted in the production of a condition called sensory neuropathy. It was then discovered that intakes of approximately 500mgs of pyridoxine per day may provoke a similar neuropathy after several years of use. This neuropathy basically is a change in sensation in the fingers and toes with feelings of numbness or pins and needles and other unusual sensations. The chronic use of vitamin B6 at doses of less than 500mgs per day for up to six years have not resulted in neuropathy. Interestingly, compared with medically prescribed drugs this side effect of neuropathy is usually reversible on the discontinuation of the pyridoxine. In some practices it has been found that the supplemental use of niacin and vitamin C with vitamin B12 injections had accelerated this reversibility of the vitamin B6 neuropathy.

Another anecdotal and poorly substantiated side effect is that of a dependency state. This consists of extremely transient nervousness and tremor on sudden withdrawal of vitamin B6 supplements. Anecdotes of withdrawal depression occurring should be disregarded.

Very minor side effects which can be a nuisance should not be cause to cease treatment — mild allergy reactions to thiamine (vitamin B1), a flushing in the skin or tingling sensation from nicotinic acid (vitamin B3) and wind or loose bowels with intestinal cramps from too much vitamin C. Vitamin E may increase the anti-clotting effects of drugs such as warfarin and so should not be used when oral anticoagulants are being administered.

The doses of nutrients in Chapter 10 are generally regarded as extremely safe by most medical scientists working in this clinical field. Any side effects are unusual, minimal, reversible and usually disappear on reduction of the dose. Do seek the advice of a doctor or therapist trained in nutritional and environmental medicine.

Tacit medical approval of megavitamin therapy

An article published in the *Australian Doctor* Journal in 1989 revealed that approximately 40% of doctors now accept chronic fatigue syndrome as an organic illness and 77% believe that there is an organic cause for it. It was revealed in this study that methods of treatment were varied and in many cases innovative, but with several outstanding similarities. Of 122 respondents to a survey (chosen at random), 56% of doctors stated that they offered supportive counselling. 44% said that they gave vitamin therapy usually in intravenous form. The vitamins most often used were vitamin C, B12, B-complex, minerals and calcium. Other forms of diet therapy including elimination diets were used by up to 25% of doctors surveyed. The next most frequent recommendation was rest of various degrees and this was advised by 25% of respondents. Drug therapy was used by only 20% of the doctors.

The salient feature about this survey conducted by Dr Andrew Lloyd at the University of New South Wales is that nearly one half of the doctors randomly selected for the study were administering a form of nutritional medicine known as orthomolecular therapy. It is indeed fortunate for the general public and patients who are suffering from the chronic fatigue syndrome that so many doctors now have, through practical experience, confirmed the usefulness of these methods in clinical practice.

The powerful prejudices held by medical academics in this country against vitamin and megavitamin therapy certainly don't appear to have filtered through and influenced the practitioner treating sick patients. The acceptance of megavitamin therapy by the community and nearly 50% of medical practitioners bears a strong resemblance to the acceptance of penicillin and aspirin into medicine without the usual double blind trials.

Much more research work needs to be done in the area of nutrients and the chronic fatigue syndrome. It should be funded by government research in a university with the foresight to create a faculty of natural medicine.

CHAPTER EIGHT

Body pollution detoxification

The main aim of any treatment programme should be to raise the patient's vitality. This is basically what doctors of natural medicine have been doing for the last one hundred years. In the time of Hippocrates, over two thousand years ago, and also in ancient China, the role of the healer and physician was to cleanse the body. Many techniques have been devised for such 'cleansing' and 'raising of the vitality' with some being more popular and effective than others.

These concepts of detoxification, cleansing and elevation of vitality are foreign to most Western-trained doctors. They are also concepts that most of the population are either unaware of or ignore. Although the increasing pollution of our air, water and food has rung alarm bells in some sections of modern society, most people don't realise the full impact that even small quantities of pollution have on the delicate machinery within the body's cells.

Naturopaths have been talking for hundreds of years about the elimination of poisonous products in the system. These poisonous products include not only the toxic substances we receive from the external environment but also the elimination of toxic products produced by the body's metabolism itself. The new field of environmental medicine encompasses all of those factors in the environment which impinge on our health including chemicals, pesticides, herbicides, heavy metals, household chemicals, positive air ions, electromagnetic smog, air, pollution etc.

However, the concept of the large bowel being a part of the environment and having the ability to produce highly toxic substances because of the huge number of bacteria, fungi and micro-organisms present in it, is something that is only becoming more appreciated over the last couple years. According to the doctrines of natural medicine and healing, those pollutants — or toxins as they are commonly called — must be eliminated from the body and therefore reduce the total toxin load. As a part of a detoxification programme, one of the major approaches to treatment involves reducing exposure to various toxins, chemicals, allergens, drugs, food additives and the multitudinous collection of chemicals present in everyday household and workplace.

Detoxification also involves the elimination of toxins from within the body itself. This includes cleansing of the bowel and the placement in the bowel of micro-organisms that are beneficial to the host. Bacteria, fungi and candida albicans are major allergens present in the bowel that can produce disease. The removal of heavy metals, such as mercury and lead, may be necessary, and this entails the use of chelation therapy. Chelation is the use of an intravenous agent which binds to heavy metals in the tissues, making them more water soluble and carrying them to the kidneys for excretion. As an integral part of a detoxification programme the use of antioxidant nutrients including vitamins A, C, selenium and zinc is mandatory.

These early steps in a treatment programme confer upon the sick person a degree of improved health without the use of toxic, synthetic drugs, drugs have the potential for symptom relief but disease promotion.

It must be remembered that although detoxification is a most essential step in the initial treatment of any disease, it may actually aggravate some of the symptoms of disease in the early stages. This probably occurs as a consequence of a change in metabolism and if there is sluggish functioning of the kidneys and liver, waste products may not be eliminated efficiently and quickly enough. These wastes form free radicals which have the ability to damage the cells and tissues of the body. This can further aggravate the disease process. Free radicals can be blocked by the use of adequate antioxidant nutrients. These antioxidant nutrients are discussed in Chapter 5 on free radical disease and antioxidants.

To improve the effects of a detoxification and antioxidant programme, the patient must be encouraged to drink plenty of fresh, pure water and to pass at least two well-formed bowel actions each day. A good detoxification programme therefore includes the stimulation of the organs of elimination including the kidneys, liver, bowel, lungs and lymphatics. This stimulation can be achieved with the appropriate use of exercise, herbal medicines, homeopathic medicines, diet, saunas and, if necessary, intravenous vitamin C.

In the chronic fatigue syndrome it appears that the nervous system, endocrine system, immune system, liver and lymphatics are the major organs under stress. It is therefore important to provide nutrients in the form of foods and herbal remedies for the various systems to enable them to recover sufficiently. Once these organs are functioning normally again, other treatments seem to have a better effect.

Detoxification of the liver

The liver is one of the largest organs in the body and it has many functions. The liver produces proteins, antibodies, anticoagulant factors, bile for fat digestion and it is intrinsically tied up with the metabolism of glucose for energy.

One of its major roles is as a detoxifying or cleansing factory. The action of the liver as a detoxifying organ is to make potentially toxic chemicals more water soluble so that they can be excreted in the bile or through the kidneys. These water soluble chemicals are produced by enzyme action in the cells of the liver and all of these enzymes are dependent on minerals, trace elements and vitamins acting as co-factors to make them work. The liver is responsible for the detoxification of chemicals obtained from the environment as well as those produced by the body's metabolism. An overload of chemicals arriving at the liver from the environment, including the environment within the large bowel, may excessively stress the liver. An excess of alcohol or tobacco, an anaesthetic, antibiotic drugs or even a mild viral infection may be the straw that breaks the camel's back. As a consequence, the liver begins to function in a sluggish manner in all respects. Until detoxification and elimination in the large bowel is improved suboptimal liver function is sure to retard a patient's recovery.

A number of liver enhancing treatments are available in natural medicine to achieve better function. Briefly, the main liver treatments include the stimulation of bile production and bile flow, the protection of the liver cells from free radical damage and inflammation, the stimulation of the repair mechanism of the liver and the activation and modulation of the immune system cells in the liver known as the Kupffer cells. Briefly we mention here some of the various nutrients and herbs that act on the liver nutritionally.

Methionine is a sulphur containing amino acid that helps to prevent the accumulation of fat globules in the cells of the damaged liver. In fact, methionine can actually assist in the mobilisation of fat accumulation in the liver cells. To stimulate bile production and bile flow herbs such as the globe artichoke, dandelion root, greater celandine and golden seal have been scientifically demonstrated to be particularly useful. Carnitine is a complex molecule formed from the amino acid lysine. To form carnitine from lysine, it is interesting to note that vitamin C is essential for the converting enzymes. Carnitine is essential for the transport of free fatty acids into the mitochondria or power houses of the cells. Once carnitine has delivered the free fatty acids to the mitochondria of every cell in our body, the mitochondria can convert the fatty acids into carbon dioxide, water and energy. This is the basic way in which energy is produced for every cell, tissue and organ of the system. Therefore a lack of lysine, vitamin C, carnitine, essential fatty acids or enzymes involved in these processes may result in a reduction of energy production by the cells. If this occurs in the liver then we see a winding down of liver function and a patient showing signs of liver sluggishness.

Naturally occurring substances have been found in plants which actually protect the liver and cells from chemical and radiation damage. Milk thistle seeds, Catechin and dimethylglycine all protect the liver to some degree against chemical toxins. Milk thistle seeds and a herb called skullcap have an anti-inflammatory effect on the liver and reduce the inflammatory damage caused by viruses and chemicals. Licorice root and again milk thistle seeds help to regenerate a damaged liver. The liver is also a very important immune organ and it contains immune cells called Kupffer cells that are stimulated into performing immunological functions in the liver by such herbs as echinacea, wild indigo and golden seal. The use of a combination of these various herbs is invaluable in patients who have had acute viral infections, acute intoxications including alcohol, drugs and chemicals or even a very poor diet.

Improving lymphatic function

The lymphatic system of the body consists of hundreds of thousands of very fine tubes, much finer than arteries and veins, which carry waste material from tissues and organs back to a much larger tube called the thoracic duct which drains the lymph and all of its wastes into the blood vessels as they enter the heart.

The lymphatics also carry lymphocytes or white blood cells and they pass through the lymph nodes, liver and spleen where important immune system functioning is carried out. The very fine tubules that carry the lymph can very easily be blocked resulting in a build-up of waste materials in many tissues and organs of the body. For many decades natural medicine specialists and naturopaths have advocated various techniques to improve lymphatic flow. The stimulation of lymph flow and the prevention of lazy lymph vessels remains an essential part of the natural detoxification process.

One of the main methods by which lymph flow can be stimulated is muscle action including exercise, yoga, stretching and rebounding. Massage is also another effective way of moving lymph through the tissues. Lymphatic massage is a special technique learned by specialist masseurs for the treatment of various conditions including acne, chronic pain and arthritis. The elevation of extremities and even the partial inversion of the whole body is another way of draining lymph and its wastes. Total inversion (i.e. with the head down and the legs up) for example standing on one's head, is not recommended. Hydrotherapy and spa jets also provide a means of massage to the tissues and all of these methods are generally fairly safe and without untoward side effects. In fact, some of them can be fun and enjoyed by all the members of the family.

Exercise itself is a form of lymphatic massage and if it's overdone in the unfit individual can result in a stirring up of toxins in the body and a general feeling of unwellness, fatigue and perhaps even nausea after the exercise has been completed.

Vigorous exercise and massage programmes should be avoided in preference to some gentler exercise such as stretching and yoga. As part of the lymphatic stimulation, improvement of spleen function and blood flow to the spleen is important. It has been shown that the herbs barberry and golden seal can stimulate these functions of the spleen which may then result in the enhancement of its immunological activities.

Detoxification by improving lymphatic flow

1. Massage by special technique called lymphatic drainage.
2. Elevation of the affected parts and elevation of the foot of the bed.
3. Exercise such as stretching, yoga, tai chi and rebounding.
4. Spa jets and hydrotherapy including water aerobics.
5. Herbal therapies especially for patients with enlarged lymph nodes (glands). These herbs include marigold, cleavers, poke root, fenugreek, wild indigo and queen's delight.

Fasting

The prevention or treatment of certain diseases by abstaining from foods for a defined time and under optimal conditions has been practised for thousands of years. Fasting is actually defined as the total abstinence from all food and drink, except water, for a specific period of time; it differs from starvation which means death or dying from a lack of food.

Many illnesses and diseases have been treated successfully by the use of properly controlled fasts and patients suffering the chronic fatigue syndrome actually benefit from fasting. This suggests that foods, chemicals or their metabolites may be precipitating the fatigue syndrome.

People in both the east and the west have performed fasting as a religious observance from ancient times. Healers and physicians from these periods observed the therapeutic effect of religious fasts and adopted them into practice. Fasting was practised by the followers of Brahmanism and was adopted later by the Buddhists in India. In the fifteenth century, Buddhism was introduced to Japan and fasting was further refined into a Buddhist rite. Buddhism and its fasting rite then spread throughout Japan. It is interesting to observe that in India, fasting is an acceptable method of treating illness and the Japanese have probably done more scientific and medical investigation and research into fasting than any other country. Fasting therapies have also been exhaustively studied in the USSR. Published data in western scientific literature is scarce.

Voluntary or involuntary fasting has been a way of life since primordial humans first began to scrounge around for food. Athanaeus, the second century Greek physician, claimed that fasting 'cures diseases, dries up bodily humours, puts demons to flight, gets rid of impure thoughts, makes the mind clearer and the heart purer, the body sanctified, and raises man to the throne of God'. Moses and Jesus fasted for forty days to bring on divine revelations, Tolstoy and his contemporaries in Russia fasted to divert the mind from materialistic concerns and 'to give joy to the soul', American Indians fasted to induce visions and dreams, and colonial New Englanders fasted to discipline themselves, save food, time and money. These are powerful testimonies to a very simple therapy and in modern day terms we can summarise this by saying that therapeutic fasting generally improves the well-being of the person fasting.

The Japanese, Russians and, more recently, the Americans have discovered fasting therapy can bring relief to patients suffering from psychosomatic disorders, gynaecological disease and even psychiatric disorders. They have been directing their attention not only to the clinical effects of fasting but also to identifying the neurological, physiological, hormonal, metabolic and psychological changes in the body which can be scientifically measured.

It has been found that patients who have some insight into

their disease and an active desire for improvement generally benefit most from fasting — sometimes dramatically — including large numbers of schizophrenic patients who have now been studied in the east and the west. This also tends to support the accumulating evidence which shows that schizophrenia is a chemical disorder of the nervous system caused primarily from food derived chemical substances, or aggravated by these metabolites.

A common symptom running through nearly all physical, psychiatric and psychosomatic disease is that of fatigue. The postulation is that if the cause of the early fatigue is discovered the development of the physical or mental disease may be prevented.

Why fasting should work is unknown. The Japanese and Russian scientists studying fasting believe that while it leads to a state of acute exhaustion, fasting actually serves as a powerful stimulus to subsequent recuperation. In the chronic fatigue syndrome, providing the patient is not overloaded with heavy metals and high levels of pesticide and herbicide residues, fasting one day a week or up to four days a month definitely helps in their recovery. Improvement generally occurs on each and every subsequent fast. Fasting ensures total rest of the digestive tract and the central nervous system. Large quantities of energy are required for the functioning of the digestive system, the production of its enzymes, absorbtion of food and the assimilation of food into the body. Simply giving the digestive tract a rest helps reduce the requirements for energy.

It is also known that the gastrointestinal tract and digestive systems relay messages back to the central nervous system when food is being processed. These relay messages may actually slow down some of the functions of the nervous system and induce a state of sleepiness or fatigue. Furthermore, food allergens have been shown to cross the gastrointestinal tract barrier and enter the bloodstream, causing allergies. These allergies are often associated with a severe state of tiredness and lethargy, apathy and fatigue. Hence, a fast rests the gastrointestinal tract, the central nervous system and possibly every other tissue and organ in the body. This rest may help to normalise function.

It has also been suggested that the acidosis or increased acid in the blood provoked by fasting and its compensation reflect a mobilisation of detoxifying defence mechanisms which probably play an important role in the total metabolic process. There are quite a number of processes which occur in the body's physiology during fasting. Acidosis occurs which increases over a period of time and then decreases due to the body's ability to compensate. Proteins are mobilised from stores in the body and enter the blood in the first week of fasting. Enzyme levels also increase in the blood and tissues, as does cholesterol. However, the initial rise in cholesterol falls if fasting continues.

Interestingly, serotonin, a chemical derived from the amino acid tryptophan in the diet and which is responsible for the sleep-wake cycle actually increases in the early stages of a fast and then falls below pre-fast levels when the fast is broken. This may be one of the mechanisms by which the chronic fatigue syndrome actually improves after a series of fasts — the level of serotonin being set lower than it had prior to the fasting treatment. Another interesting neurotransmitter change is the level of catecholamine metabolites. The catecholamines include adrenaline and noradrenaline which are the fight and flight response hormones secreted by the adrenal glands. These catecholamines are also produced in the central nervous system and are responsible for increased alertness, reduced fatigue levels and generally an increase in the state of anxiety symptoms. These catecholamine metabolites rise during a fast and remain set at higher values after re-feeding.

The changes relating to the central nervous system, including the brain and nerves, are observed in the electroencephalogram (EEG). The EEG measures the brainwave activity in the form of electrical impulses which can be converted by the EEG machine to a graph. The waves that are seen on the graph are classified according to their frequency. The slow alpha waves are extremely prominent after a fast. These are the waves that are responsible for the relaxed meditative state. It has been shown that the beta waves of thirteen to twenty cycles per second — that is, faster waves than the alpha waves — are reduced significantly during and after fasting therapy. These beta waves are the waves responsible for anxiety states. It can be seen therefore that definite changes occur which can be measured during and after fasts and these changes may help to explain the clinical improvements seen in patients who undergo fasting therapy.

Incidently, these measurable EEG changes persist for up to

3 months after the cessation of the fast.

There are certain conditions under which fasting therapy should not be undertaken and these include an abnormality of the heart on the ECG or heart disease, pre-disposition to thrombosis, past history of a heart block or other serious disease, cancers of all forms, severe blood disorders, pregnancy, active lung disease except asthma and severely disturbed, unmotivated or psychotic patients. The fast should be broken if abnormal heart rhythms occur, rapid heart rates, rapid pulse rates, abdominal pains, persistent and severe hunger or a disturbance to a patient's psychological and mental state occurs.

Of the disorders listed below, 87% of 380 patients greatly benefitted from the fasting therapy. Interestingly, in this study, it was shown that the long-term results of fasting therapy also showed very similar effects. Excellent results in the long-term follow-up of these patients occurred in 22% and good results in 65% of patients. Even more interesting is the fact that those patients who did not benefit from fasting therapy immediately gained moderate clinical improvement up to three months after the fasting. This suggests that fasting therapy may not, in the short term, always produce results but some mechanism may continue to operate to the patient's benefit after the fast. The chronic neurasthenia syndrome mentioned in the disorders included below is very similar clinically to the chronic fatigue syndrome and was one of the synonyms used for the chronic fatigue syndrome before its official recognition.

Disorders studied in fasting therapy

1. Migraine
2. Diabetes
3. Hypertension
4. Chronic neurasthenia
5. Irritable bowel syndrome
6. Arthritis
7. Anxiety and depression
8. Asthma
9. Hyperventilation syndrome

There are some basic rules that must be followed during a fast, whether it be one day a week or a four day a month fast.

For the inexperienced, it is certainly not recommended that anything longer than a four day fast once a month be attempted. The fasting person must be out of bed and active during the fast. Hunger must cease within a short period of time. The fasting ideally must be absolute — that is, there should be no food intake whatsoever. Fasting means the absence of all food and the use of water only. If juices are used during a fast then it is not regarded as a true fast but fresh fruit or vegetable juices, if diluted 50% with water, are suggested if a water fast is too difficult. The fruits and vegetables used in juicing should be organically grown and as free of pesticides and herbicides as possible.

Yoga, stretching or walking are ideal exercises to be performed during the fast and encourage the bowels to remain active. Hunger should diminish by the second or third day of the fast and at no times during the fast should it be severe. If it is, then the fast should be broken. At least two litres of purified and filtered water should be consumed daily. A daily weighing should be performed. It has been suggested that bowel cleansing enemas are of benefit. However, if the bowel has been treated properly prior to the fasting therapy and lactobacillus, bifidobacteria combinations used prior to the fast, the bowel should be reasonably clean. Drugs and medications that are not absolutely necessary should be reduced or stopped completely prior to the fast under appropriate medical supervision.

Smoking is also strictly forbidden, and the avoidance of other air pollutants is strongly advised because of the increased sensitivity to inhaled odours and smells whilst fasting.

Fasting should be broken gently by the introduction of diluted fruit and vegetable juices and lightly steamed vegetables for the first few meals. Certainly heavy grains, animal proteins and dairy products must be avoided in the early stage of the 'break fast' and avoided completely if allergies to them are diagnosed.

Diseases responding to fasting therapies

1. Headache and migraine
2. Diabetes

3. Hypertension
4. Gout
5. Chronic neurasthenia (now called chronic fatigue syndrome)
6. Inflammatory disorders
7. Irritable bowel syndrome
8. Epilepsy
9. Obesity
10. Hypertensive heart disease
11. Hyperlipidaemia
12. Hypercholesterolaemia
13. Mild congestive cardiac failure
14. Low HDL cholesterol
15. Pancreatitis
16. Arthritis
17. Pain syndromes
18. Food intolerance
19. Food allergies
20. Glomerulonephritis
21. Autoimmune diseases
22. DDT poisoning (**Caution** — Chemicals may be mobilised from fat tissues during fasting)
23. PCB intoxication (**Caution** — Chemicals may be mobilised from fat tissues during fasting)
24. Psoriasis, eczema
25. Varicose ulcers
26. Depression and anxiety
27. Asthma
28. Hyperventilation syndrome

All of the above diseases have been scientifically evaluated and show a definite response to fasting therapy.

The cleansing diet

The dietary programme and food composition of the patient with the chronic fatigue syndrome represents a complicated aspect of their highly individualised treatment programme. Inappropriate eating habits over the whole of a lifetime, or for that matter a few weeks or months, are implied in the majority of degenerative diseases facing modern westerners. These inappropriate eating habits and nutrient depleted foods such as junk foods, fast foods and processed foods, account for a wide range of deficiencies and/or excesses which eventually lead to a weakening of the organism and finally a disease state.

Although many people with the chronic fatigue syndrome believe that they are consuming a well-balanced diet of good foods, on further questioning they are often found to be consuming empty calorie, high fat content, high sugar content products for up to 30% of their total food intake. Even CFS sufferers who eat a wide variety of foods that are fresh and unprocessed cannot assume that they are receiving optimum concentrations of nutrients required for their best health. It is under such conditions of imbalance and borderline deficiency states that unresolved viral infections and stress will result in damage albeit reversible to the main systems affected, that is nervous, hormonal and immune.

For the great majority of people with chronic fatigue syndrome and other nutritionally responsive diseases, dietary changes, corrections and nutritional manipulation will involve major lifestyle changes.

The practical aim of therapeutic nutrition is to help to bring the person back into a balanced state of body chemistry for the available dietary energy to be used for homeostasis and the healing process, and not for the fight against disease. To achieve this, a balanced diet containing all of the important nutrients is essential. In industrialised western society, it is virtually impossible for an optimally balanced nutritional programme to be attained without the use of some additional supplementation. This has been scientifically verified.

The three main killer diseases in western society are cancer, heart disease and stroke and it has been scientifically and medically demonstrated that these diseases are caused by a poor diet. It has also been demonstrated beyond any doubt whatsoever that people with these diseases and many of the other degenerative diseases in our western society have multiple nutritional deficiency states. The standard Australian diseases of heart disease, cancer and stroke, diabetes, arthritis and inflammatory bowel disease are strongly related to the standard Australian diet.

The issue of supplementation in the diet is covered in other chapters of this book.

Aims of the cleansing and rejuvenation dietary programme

1. The replenishment of nutrients that are in short supply or deficient in fresh, natural, whole, unprocessed foods including raw vegetables, salads and juices.
2. To reduce the toxic, metabolic and chemical load on the nervous, immune and hormone systems.
3. To accelerate the detoxification processes and mechanisms in the bowel, liver and kidneys.
4. To provide antioxidant-dense foods that protect the cells and tissues of the body against highly reactive free radicals.
5. To reduce the energy requirements of the digestive system including the liver, pancreas and small intestine by decreasing the complexity of foods eaten, including animal proteins.

    Note — Some metabolic types may do better on small regular snacks of animal protein. This is discussed elsewhere under metabolic types.

6. To reduce the toxic load, not only of chemicals but also artificial stimulants such as sugar, alcohol, tea, coffee, chocolate, cola drinks and of course drugs including tobacco, marijuana, cocaine etc.
7. To restrict, or completely eliminate if possible, the following substances which have been demonstrated scientifically to retard the healing process:-

Cortisone	Some anti-inflammatory drugs
Anti-depressant drugs	
Anti-anxiety drugs	The oral contraceptive pill
Coffee	Aspirin
Beta-blocking drugs	
Sleeping medications including barbiturates and other hypnotics	

8. To encourage the use of raw fruit and vegetable juices diluted 50% in purified water to provide living enzymes, vitamins, minerals, trace elements and probably other life-

giving healing factors that science has yet to isolate and define.
9. To eliminate added salt to the diet.
10. To eliminate all additives including artificial colourings, flavourings, emulsifiers, preservatives, synthetic antioxidants.
11. No fried foods are allowed and fats and oils should be greatly restricted. This does not apply to the essential fatty acids which may be added to the nutritional programme as supplements. These essential fatty acids include the EPA of fish oil and evening primrose oil.
12. To encourage grazing on six to eight small meals per day rather than two or three mail meals.

Cleansing fruits

Natural medicine specialists the world over have learnt that the following fruits are very cleansing:-

Apples	Paw paw (Papaya)
Avocado	Pineapple
Cranberries	Watermelon
Grapes	

Paw paw (papaya) is an excellent fruit because it contains high concentrations of digestive enzymes and it is very easily digested and assimilated. Oranges and lemons are also extremely useful in a general cleansing programme and they also contain a good natural source of vitamin C and the extremely important bioflavonoids.

Cleansing vegetables

The following vegetables, providing they are fresh and organically grown, are also regarded as very useful cleansing and healing foods:

Asparagus	Celery Dandelion leaves
Avocado	Green peppers
Beetroot and its leaves	Horseradish (fresh)
Carrots	Lentils (partially sprouted)

Lettuce
Onions
Parsley
Potatoes (in their skins)

Spinach and silverbeet
Turnip tops
Watercress

Of course if one is sensitive or allergic to any of these fruits or vegetables they must be avoided.

Nuts and seeds, provided they are not consumed in large quantities, are also helpful during a cleansing, detoxification programme. All nuts, except peanuts, providing they are fresh and not rancid are safe. Sesame seeds, pumpkin seeds and sunflower seeds are highly nutritious and fresh sesame seed paste is a good substitute spread for butter and margarine. Garlic, parsley and lemon juice can be added and blended to give it extra flavour.

Sprouts made from alfalfa, mung beans, lentils and clover are highly nutritious and contain living enzymes.

Drinks include 10 to 12 glasses of purified water every day and herbal teas are highly recommended. These include dandelion tea, peppermint tea, rosehips, chamomile and lemongrass.

Organically grown brown rice, millet and buckwheat are the most appropriate grains as they don't provoke allergic reactions as frequently as wheat, barley, rye and oats. In fact, the gluten containing grains — wheat, barley, rye and oats are common offending foods in the patient with the chronic fatigue syndrome. Whether it is the gluten or gliadin or other components of these grains causing the fatigue, lethargy and weakness is unknown. However, it's wise to avoid these grains and dairy products including milk, butter, cream, cheese and yoghurt, at least in the early stages of treatment.

Meat and animal proteins are generally banned completely in a strict detoxification and cleansing programme. However, animal protein in the form of yoghurt and fish may be permitted if the metabolic make-up of the individual warrants it. Even small quantities of red meat may be allowed in patients who are sensitive to grains, have difficulty gaining weight, and who generally feel better on a higher protein diet.

Other foods that are permitted in smaller quantities include rye bread, non-fat cottage cheese, stewed fruits in small quantities, boiled or poached free-range eggs, olive oil (maximum of 1 tablespoon per day), fresh fish (no other seafood including shellfish), lambs fry, unsterilised yoghurt (unsweetened and unflavoured), all types of nuts, fresh and raw (exclude roasted, salted nuts and peanuts), chives, marjoram, thyme, sage, oregano, cummin, coriander, ginger, cinnamon, cloves, cardamon, horseradish and pollen.

From practical experience with hundreds of patients suffering from fatigue and the chronic fatigue syndrome, the most effective way of eating is through the macrobiotic approach. The macrobiotic diet and modifications of it cannot be covered in detail in a single chapter. It is recommended that if you are serious about consuming the best possible diet for the chronic fatigue syndrome you should attend macrobiotic cooking classes and refer to some of the references at the end of this book.

In brief, we obtain our energy from the sun through the foods that we eat. The various organic nutrients in our foods contain the energy information from the sun for our utilisation and it is basically through foods, nutrients and nutrient substances that we can improve the health of every living cell and tissue in the human body. The results of a cleansing, detoxification and rejuvenation diet do not occur immediately but may take three to six weeks before they are seen. What happens after that initial improvement is up to the individual. Nutrition and diet are with us for life — we eat food until the day we die. The way we feel is directly related to what we eat — a little self discipline is far less hampering than chronic ill health.

Colon therapy

The colon is another name for the large intestine. The large intestine is the organ which receives the remains of the food that has been eaten and digested in the small intestine. This food waste is referred to as the faeces which are eliminated via the colon and rectum and anus. In fact, the colon is part of an empty tube that begins at the mouth, passes through the gullet, stomach, small intestine then the large intestine and exits through the anus. This hollow tube is twisted and in places very narrow (intestines) or very swollen (stomach) and receives tubes from various glands including the liver and the pancreas. It may be regarded as a part of the external environment. Hence the contents of the colon are a part of the external environment and the waste material (faeces) is only temporarily carried there until it is expelled through the process of defecation.

The environment of the colon is extremely active biologically. It was once thought that the colon was simply an organ for the passage and removal of faeces. However, it is known that water is actively absorbed from the faeces in the colon into the circulation and many organic and inorganic substances are produced by the billions of bacteria berthed in the faeces. These substances can be absorbed through the bowel and pass into the liver via the bloodstream where they are meant to be inactivated. The types of microorganisms that make up the faeces determine the state of health of the individual. The correct type of bacteria are conducive to good health whereas the incorrect bacteria can actually contribute to poor health and may even cause overt disease.

Colon cleansing therapy has been used for centuries in natural medicine and it dates back to the time of the ancient Chinese. The highly controversial nature of colon therapy which persists until this day will eventually be quashed in the light of recent scientific evidence. Despite what many people believe as a crude and unclean form of therapy, colon treatments are relatively simple, safe, inexpensive and very effective. Colon treatment is more than just a simple enema or irrigation. It generally involves dietary changes, herbal medicines, fluid therapy, recolonisation procedures, all dependent on appropriate diagnosis of the physical, chemical and biological properties of the bowel and its faeces.

Types of colon therapy

1. Plain or herbal enemas
2. Colonic irrigation
3. Coffee enemas (not recommended)
4. Colectomy (surgical removal of the colon)
5. Recolonisation of the colon
6. Specific dietary fibre
7. Improving blood flow

A majority of sufferers of the chronic fatigue syndrome note that prior to their illness they had suffered from a viral or bacterial infection. Should the infection have involved the gastrointestinal tract with flu-like symptoms, abdominal pains, diarrhoea, nausea and perhaps vomiting the possibility of a disturbance in the balance of microorganisms in the bowel is very high. Treatment with antibiotics for the initial infection can further grossly disrupt the normal bacteria in the bowel and may even result in the overgrowth of fungi, yeasts and a particularly damaging organism — candida albicans.

Candida albicans is responsible for the disease known as oral thrush, an infection which consists of a creamy white irritating discharge from the vagina, nappy rash in babies, skin rashes in adults and white plaque-like lesions on the gums of the mouth. Candida albicans is discussed in more detail in another section.

For centuries it has been known by lay people and healers, doctors of natural medicine and even orthodox physicians, that the large intestine plays a major role in a wide range of diseases. In fact this range is probably greater than most people appreciate. 'Have the bowels opened, 'cleanse the bowels' and other similar phrases have resounded in the major healing centres and hospitals throughout the world since antiquity.

The health spas and centres of Europe emphasise fasting, juices and aperients as part of their basic programmes for the treatment of arthritis, migraine headaches and chronic unwellness. Other diseases directly related to the diet and colon health include diverticulosis, irritable bowel syndrome, rectal polyps, appendicitis and even carcinoma (cancer) of the colon and rectum.

Colonic health is dependent on fibre in the diet and even minor changes to the amount or type of fibre can have a significant effect on the health of the bowel. The removal of fibre from the diet is associated with a large number of diseases including those of the large bowel mentioned above. These fibre deficiency associated disorders include high cholesterol levels, varicose veins, diabetes, gall stones, coronary heart disease and perhaps even stroke. Hence, plant food or dietary fibre as it's more commonly known is intrinsically woven into the health, not only of the gastrointestinal tract, but of the nation as a whole.

The internal environment and metabolism of the contents of the colon is dependent not only on dietary factors but also the types of bacteria and other microorganisms present. In the following table we see the various influences on bowel health.

Factors determining the health of the internal environment of the colon

1. Allergenic and sensitising foods
2. Pesticide, herbicide and other xenobiotic chemicals in the diet
3. Abnormal pancreatic, liver and gall bladder functions
4. Poor quality or deficient dietary fibre (plant foods)
5. Disturbances in immunological function
6. Abnormal microorganisms in the faeces
7. Psychological stress factors
8. Inadequate exercise

Food allergies and foods to which a patient is sensitive may result in the fatigue syndrome. However, allergenic foods can produce other problems including a suppression of liver, pancreatic and gall bladder functioning and an inhibition of intestinal enzymes also. The result is the incomplete digestion and breakdown of food components and their passage through the gastrointestinal tract undigested, resulting in direct entry of unassimilated food into the large intestine. It is here in the large intestine that these undigested food proteins, carbohydrates and fats are acted on by the microorganisms and bacteria in the bowel to produce a wide range of toxic substances including indoles, skatoles, spermine and putrescine. These compounds are absorbed through the bowel wall and enter into the bloodstream with effects that are potentially damaging. These toxic organic molecules have been shown to have an effect on liver function, immune function and the activity of the central nervous system. They may also interfere with the body's hormones.

These chemicals together with toxic amines can also cause local tissue damage which may explain why approximately 90% of patients with the chronic fatigue syndrome also suffer from abdominal bloating, intestinal gas and disturbances in bowel function generally. Diarrhoea may also occur in 40% of patients and up to 65% of patients will complain of abdominal pains and halitosis (bad breath). These symptoms can often be easily corrected by a change in diet, the removal of food allergens and correcting abnormal food combining patterns. The avoidance of combining foods such as proteins and carbohydrates, fruits and vegetables, and grains with citrus fruits relieves abdominal symptoms in more than half of patients suffering. It has been shown that the damaged lining of the bowel due to some of these chemicals and toxic substances will result in an increase in permeability of the bowel membrane. This allows the toxins, bacterial products and food components to enter the bloodstream directly. The blood then presents these unusual components to the liver which has to handle the increased load of toxins and allergens for detoxification.

Optimal pancreatic, liver and gall bladder function are very important for the health of the individual from the perspective of proper digestion, absorption and assimilation of nutrients. The adequate digestion and breakdown of food in the upper small intestine is also important from another point of view. That is, this process if adequate will reduce the load of undigested protein, carbohydrate, fat and other foodstuffs from entering the large intestine as discussed above.

Detoxification implants

It is extremely pertinent when discussing environmental medicine to keep in mind the internal environment of the large bowel. The health of this organ and its environment has been ignored by modern medicine. However, recent research shows that the large intestine is a dynamic organ and its contents may play a major role in the wellness of the individual. The aspects of toxin production by abnormal bacteria, fungi and spores the effect the liver and immune system are discussed in the section on toxemia in the bowel.

For centuries people around the world have used some form of fermented food in their diet ranging from miso, kefir and various yoghurts. This fermentation process has been a means by which foods can be preserved in a healthy, nutritious and tasty state. Of great importance to the diets of many cultures are foods fermented with various bacilli (bacteria) which convert milk sugar or lactose to lactic acid. These lacto fermenting bacteria are known generally as lactobacilli. Recent documented medical evidence has proven that the lactobacilli are not just simply symbiotic organisms that live in harmony with humankind but that they are actually bacteria which are important in the prevention and in the possible of some major diseases such as Crohn's disease and ulcerative colitis. The actual culturing of milk and dairy products not only preserves the foods but it actually retains all of the original nutrients including proteins, fatty acids, vitamins, minerals and trace elements. It also converts some of the nutrients into more bioavailable forms and breaks others down into simpler compounds.

Our first exposure to this family of bacteria is through breast milk. Breastfeeding actually introduces lactobacillus bifidus into the gastrointestinal tract of the newborn infant. With continued breastfeeding the bifidus colonises the gut and becomes a dominant strain of bacteria in the faeces of the baby. Other bacteria of the lactobacillus family colonise the bowel and live in harmony with one another. Depending on various factors and dietary circumstances, these bacteria may be displaced by harmful organisms that are potentially toxic.

A poor diet high in sugar, alcohol drinking and the use of antibiotics either as medicines or in foodstuffs are the most common causes of a disturbed bowel flora.

It is clear that lactobacilli are important in the chronic fatigue syndrome because of reasons of infection in the bowel or the use of antibiotics. As we have seen earlier, many patients with the chronic fatigue syndrome have had a viral or bacterial infection which may or may not have been treated with an antibiotic. These events result in the development of abnormal bowel flora and it is for this reason that lactobacillus plays an important part in the recovery of health of the CFS patient. One of the most significant therapeutic effects of lactobacilli is their antibiotic properties. Lactobacilli have been shown to inhabit the growth of other micro organisms in the bowel and vagina through competition for nutrients for survival, by increasing the acidity of the vagina or bowel and by utilising the available oxygen necessary for the growth and reproduction of disease causing bacteria.

Another very interesting antibiotic-like effect of lactobacilli is their ability to prevent the attachment of other bacteria to the lining cells of the bowel wall. This prevents the attachment of and subsequent penetration of these bacteria into the system. Antibiotic and antimicrobial substances are produced by the lactobacillus family and generally maintain a healthy environment within the large intestine.

An increase in the variety of foods containing lactobacilli organisms are appearing in the marketplace in addition to the pure lactobacilli supplements available in tablet, capsule and pure powder form. In clinical practice the choice of the form of lactobacilli is extremely important. Generally the most effective form is a powder called Lactobac which contains lactobacillus acidophilus and lactobacillus bifidus. The desirable actions of the lactobacillus family can be obtained by using a combination of these two formulas. Lactobacilli are extremely fastidious in their metabolic requirements and they are significantly effected by the diet, sugars, antibiotics and alcohol. Acidophilus and bifidus are normal inhabitants of the intestine and can adapt quite readily. They generally perform most of the functions which are advantageous to the host as mentioned below. The Lactobac powder that has been studied the most in the chronic fatigue syndrome is the ideal preparation for these purposes. One teaspoon two to three times per day prior to meals for one week reduced to one teaspoon daily thereafter is sufficient in most patients to recolonise the bowel with high quality acidophilus and bifidus organisms.

Many yoghurts do not contain the correct species of lactobacillus and when they do most companies sterilise the yoghurt and render the organisms inactive. A great many products on the market containing lactobacilli, for example yoghurt and cultured milks, contain added flavourings and sugars. Sugar is inhibitory to the activity and growth of lactobacilli and therefore these products are not recommended.

Lactobacillus supplementation should always accompany and follow the use of broad spectrum antibiotics. In the chronic fatigue syndrome group of patients most of these individuals have been treated unnecessarily with antibiotics for viral infections. As a consequence the bowel flora and microorganisms are altered to the detriment of the patient. Cultures of lactobacilli should also be used for treatment of gastrointestinal disorders including viral gastroenteritis, food poisoning and severe gastrointestinal allergies. The majority of CFS patients who have symptoms in the gastrointestinal tract such as nausea, vomiting, diarrhoea, abdominal bloating, colicky abdominal pains and flatulence generally respond very well to useful preparations of lactobacilli. It is important to remember that the benefits obtained from supplementation using lactobacilli may only last for as long as the supplementation occurs. This is important in the early stages of treatment. If a chronic fatigue syndrome patient responds to lactobacilli and bifido bacteria supplementation then a maintenance supplementation programme should be continued for at least six to twelve months after commencement. Generally recommendations for lactobacilli supplementation is advised in modern environments where the food chain contains deliberately added antibiotics. Also, sugar and alcohol in the diet can often rapidly modify the type of micro-organisms in the bowel and are absolutely contraindicated in the patient with CFS.

Beneficial effects of lactobacilli

1. Produces organic and inorganic antibiotics
2. Produces anti-cancer factors
3. Has positive effects on psychological state (e.g. anti-fatigue, anti-anxiety and anti-depressant activity)
4. Neutralises cancer producing chemicals
5. Produces antiviral substances
6. Produces antifungal substances
7. Suppresses the growth of yeasts and thrush (candida)
8. Partially digests foodstuffs (e.g. milk sugar and milk proteins are broken down)
9. Synthesises certain vitamins including B-complex, folic acid, vitamin B12, vitamin K
10. May reduce the allergenicity of milk
11. Improves the quality of milk proteins
12. Destroys naturally occurring anti-nutrients in foods (e.g. phytate, antitrypsins.)
13. May reduce serum cholesterol
14. Detoxification of metabolites in liver disease
15. Reduces bowel symptoms of gastrointestinal allergies (e.g. pain, bloating, flatulence)

The family of lactobacilli have the ability to produce organic and inorganic antibiotic like substances and acids which inhibit or prohibit the growth and replication of other species of bacteria in the large intestine and vagina. Many of the pathogenic bacteria in the large bowel are inhibited by such antibiotics as acidophilin, acidolin and lactocidin. These antibiotics can suppress the activity of pathogenic bacteria that are responsible for food poisoning, gastroenteritis, abscesses, skin disease and even the organisms that cause typhus and cholera.

It has been demonstrated that abnormal bacteria and viruses can persist in the bowel of a chronic fatigue syndrome patient for more than twelve months. If this is the case and these bacteria have the ability to either produce toxin or, more seriously, to produce endotoxins on their own death, then the total toxic load on patients with this problem may render recovery an almost impossibility.

In women with the chronic fatigue syndrome another reservoir of abnormal bacteria, fungi and yeasts, is the vagina. Lactobacillus acidophilus is a normal constituent of the micro organisms in the vagina. Here the lactobacillus maintains a very acid environment by fermenting glucose to lactic acid. The amount of glucose in the vaginal cells is hormone dependent and the balance is aggravated by a high dietary intake of sugars. This fine balance if upset can result in the suppression of lactobacillus acidophilus with a consequent loss of vaginal acidity and the consequent overgrowth of abnormal bacteria, fungi and yeast. This is the ideal environment for the growth of the yeast candida - the organism that causes vaginal thrush. Lactobacillus acidophilus is also suppressed by broad spectrum antibiotics, and most women who suffer from thrush know of the nasty, irritating, creamy discharge that results. In fact, candida may be present in the vagina without producing a discharge and it can be partially responsible for chronic ill health.

Women have known for many decades that the use of yoghurt orally and as a vaginal douche helps to suppress the abnormal yeasts and bacteria and return the vaginal condition to normal. It has been recently shown scientifically that the introduction of lactobacillus into the vagina and bowel helps to suppress yeast infections. Hence, in the investigation of the female with the chronic fatigue syndrome, it must be remembered that not only the large intestine but the vagina can act as a harbour for abnormal micro organisisms, yeasts and candida. It may be very difficult in some cases to actually show candida and yeast growing in the vagina by normal laboratory methods. The organisms have the ability to penetrate the cells of the lining of the vagina and grow into the deeper tissues. This results in a situation where the tissues of the host eventually become sensitised or allergic to the microorganisms and antibodies to candida and yeasts are made by the host's immune system. These antibodies react also with yeasts in the diet and can cause severe allergic reactions including many of the symptoms commonly found in the chronic fatigue syndrome. To assist in controlling these problems, a product (Lactobac) containing lactobacillus and bifido bacteria organisms must be taken orally — one teaspoon of the powder mixed in water three times daily before meals, to help alter the flora in the large intestine. To correct the vaginal problems the powder can be mixed with an aqueous (water based) cream and inserted high into the vagina at night. This cream should also be applied to the outside tissues of the vagina.

Many patients with the chronic fatigue syndrome carry abnormal enteroviruses in their gastrointestinal tract. In approximately one third of patients these enteroviruses persist for twelve months or longer. Generally the bowel flora of these patients is abnormal and the use of Lactobac in these people will reconstitute the normal flora. As mentioned earlier, lactobacilli produce organic and inorganic acids which inactivate or inhibit viruses either directly or by increasing the acidity of the environment. Some workers in this field have postulated that lactobacilli themselves can produce specific anti-viral compounds. Non-specific antimicrobial substances produced by lactobacilli include hydrogen peroxide (common bleach), benzoic acid, acetic acid and lactic acid. Many other substances known to inhibit or suppress the overgrowth of bacteria, viruses and yeasts known to causes illness and disease are also secreted by lactobacilli. The environment of the large intestine, including its contents the faeces, is able to support the growth and reproduction of bacteria that both survive well in oxygen and others that are inhibited or killed in an oxygen rich environment. The great benefit of the lactobacilli is that they can survive under both oxygen-rich and oxygen depleted conditions. Under both these conditions, lactobacilli also secrete their anti-pathogenic substances. In practical terms this means that high concentrations of lactobacilli in faeces are able to suppress disease causing bacteria and harmful toxins in the large intestine.

It has been demonstrated that sufferers of the chronic fatigue syndrome have either low levels or deficiencies of one or a number of micronutrients including some of the B-group vitamins and ascorbic acid. Supplementation of these nutrients by mouth and injection is often necessary. As an adjunct to this supplementation, lactobacilli have been shown to synthesise a number of viruses including some of the B-complex and vitamin K. Lactobacilli can also increase the concentrations of B-complex vitamins in fermented milk products such as yoghurt. However, they also require a supply of B-complex vitamins for their own growth and development and dietary supplementation appears to facilitate this. Vitamin B12 is one of the more important of the B-complex vitamins in the chronic fatigue syndrome. Hence, the use of lactobacilli and injectable vitamin B12 as part of the therapeutic regime are extremely useful.

If dairy products are tolerated and the person with chronic fatigue syndrome can be shown not to be allergic to dairy foods, the safest of these foods are of course the fermented dairy products including yoghurt, kefir, acidophilis milk, bifidus milk etc. The lactic acid produced by the lactobacilli bacteria on fermentation of these products improves the digestibility and availability of the protein in the dairy foods and yields higher levels of free amino acids than the parent milk compounds. Many amino acids are of course the precursors to the neurotransmitters or nerve chemicals that transmit information from one nerve cell to another in the brain and spinal cord.

We know that chronic stress and acute viral infections can reduce the free amino acids in the bloodstream and thus decrease the availability of these amino acids for the central nervous system. This is an area that needs further investigation in the future.

Another important aspect of the digestibility of dairy products is that of lactose — milk sugar. Many people who are sensitive to dairy products react to the milk sugar (lactose) rather than have a distinct allergy to cows milk protein. This lactose intolerance is due to lack of the enzyme lactase. Lactose intolerance in individuals causes symptoms of abdominal pain, bloating and diarrhoea. However, these people are often quite tolerant of lactobacilli fermented dairy products.

In the chronic fatigue syndrome it has been demonstrated that most patients have a reactivity to cows milk proteins. Therefore in the early stages of treatment, they should avoid both fermented and unfermented dairy products. The use of pure lactobacillus acidopholis and bifidobacteria in powder form is the most efficient method of reconstituting the lactobacilli in the bowel. Even sufferers of cows milk allergy who have mild to moderate sensitivities to cows milk protein, can recommence the use of small but increasing quantities of yoghurt once their condition improves. The fermentation process produces greater acidity and this changes the structure and chemical composition of the cows milk proteins, reducing it's allergenicity. Protein digestibility and availability are often improved. This has been proven in animal studies in which the animals have shown improved weight gain.

Lactobacillus supplementation has also been shown to reduce the symptoms of gastrointestinal allergies. These gastrointestinal allergies may manifest themselves in such diverse symptoms as indigestion, symptoms mimicking peptic ulcer, bloating, abdominal pain, flatulence, diarrhoea, itchy anus, mouth ulcers and nausea. The exact mechanism by which lactobacilli accomplish these marvellous symptom relieving properties is unknown. The symbiotic relationship between this organism and humans definitely requires further studies, especially in view of the fact that it appears so useful clinically. Epidemiological studies have even indicated that the consumption of high levels of cultured dairy products may reduce the risk of cancer of the colon.

Lactobacilli also secrete anti-cancer factors. A number of enzymes secreted by unhealthy bacteria in the bowel are known to stimulate the production of carcinogens. Two of these enzymes are called nitroreductase and beta-glucuronidase. Carcinogens can be formed from nitrites and nitrates in the food that we eat. These nitrogen containing compounds are converted in the gastrointestinal tract to nitrosamines which are known carcinogens. If this conversion can be inhibited, then fewer carcinogens are manufactured in the bowel and presented to the bowel wall. Theoretically, and to some degree practically, this can be achieved. For example, the use of ascorbic acid or vitamin C in the diet can prevent the formation of nitrosamines from nitrites and nitrates. The use of lactobacillus can inhibit the activity of the abnormal bacterial enzymes which are responsible for the production of carcinogens. In fact it has been shown scientifically that after four weeks supplementation with lactobacillus acidophilis the activity of carcinogen promoting faecal enzymes can be reduced to as much as 25% of the original levels. Theoretically this may be sufficient to reduce the risk of cancer development. Blastolysins are complicated molecules which have been isolated from lactobacillus bulgaricus. These substances have been shown to have anti-tumour effects in animal cancers.

For all these reasons, lactobacilli are therefore an important aspect of total health care and the use of appropriate forms is critical to the welfare of the patient with chronic fatigue syndrome.

A further aspect of proper health maintenance and the role of the lactobacilli species of bacteria is the control of cholesterol and blood fats. There have been many conflicting studies conducted on the use of lactobacillus acidophilis and cultured dairy products in the control of blood fats and cholesterol. It could be said generally that the higher the blood concentration of cholesterol and fats (triglycerides) to commence with the greater the effect the lactobacilli have in reducing these raised levels. The reason for this is not completely understood. It has been suggested that the lactobacilli metabolise these lipids and cholesterol for their own energy and reproduction. It has also been suggested that lactobacilli may simply facilitate the excretion of cholesterol via the bowel. To reduce blood cholesterol and triglycerides using lactobacillus, high concentrations over a long period of time appear necessary.

There is no documented association between the chronic fatigue syndrome and high blood lipid levels but there certainly is a very strong suggestion that lipids peroxides and lipid free radicals are involved in the chronic fatigue syndrome. Organic reducing agents secreted by lactobacilli may, by this indirect mechanism lipid metabolism, have a beneficial effect in the CFS patient.

It has been demonstrated in liver disease including cirrhosis, chronic hepatitis and portal hypertension that the bifidus form of lactobacilli decreases a number of oxidising chemicals in the blood, including phenols and ammonia. Again, it is not known why this happens. The production of toxins in the bowel may be inhibited by lactobacillus thus reducing the total toxic load on the liver. However, this does not readily explain the situation satisfactorily. But it has been observed in patients with the chronic fatigue syndrome who have evidence of viral disease affecting the liver (abnormal liver function tests) that the well-being of the patient, and the pathology tests, improve on lactobacillus supplementation. Much more research work needs to be done on the antigenic and immunological effects of lactobacilli in these conditions. Patients with the chronic fatigue syndrome often suffer from nausea, epigastric discomfort and a tenderness of the liver. These symptoms, including the tenderness of the liver, respond to lactobacillus supplementation between three days and three weeks of commencement.

Occasionally, in approximately 20% of patients, a dieback or Herxheimer reaction occurs. This is the result of the lactobacilli inactivating or killing unwanted micro-organisms in the bowel and the subsequent release of endotoxins from the dead organisms. These substances are absorbed through the bowel wall and enter the bloodstream of the patient. Two and a half to three litres of water per day, and suitable natural cathartics to ensure optimal kidney and bowel function, reduce the severity of this problem.

Studies on the use of lactobacilli in impending hepatic encephalopathy have not been performed. Hepatic encephalopathy is a disease of the brain and nervous system due to liver failure. Although this does not occur in the chronic fatigue syndrome, it may be seen in a modified form in long term sufferers of the chronic fatigue syndrome who have developed severe liver disease as a consequence of alcoholism, drug addiction or psychotropic medication. Although these would be only a very small percentage of patients, it is mentioned here for the sake of completeness.

Lactobacilli destroy toxins in the bowel, inhibit anti-nutrients such as phytate and antitrypsin, neutralise sugars which produce gas and inhibit yeast infections.

Finally, and probably most importantly, through some unknown and definitely unappreciated mechanism, far away from the workings of the bowel and its contents, is an effect on the health of the nervous system and mind — lactobacillus supplementation results in an anti-fatigue, anti-anxiety and anti-depressant effect on the central nervous system. The liver was believed by the ancient physicians to be the sight of melancholy (sadness and depression). Melancholy comes from the Greek which means black bile. With recent information on the health of the large intestine and its faecal contents and the effects of these toxins on the liver, emotional feelings may have some of their origins in this organ of elimination.

Factors involved in the determination of the health of the internal environment of the large bowel

1. Allergenic and sensitising foods
2. Pancreatic, liver and gall bladder function (abnormal, poor quality or deficient functioning)
3. Dietary fibre (plant foods)
4. Immunological function in the wall of the bowel
5. Types of bacterial inhabitants and other micro-organisms
6. Stress
7. Exercise
8. Micronutrient supplementation (vitamin and mineral therapy)

Colon therapies

1. Plain or herbal enemas
2. Coffee enemas
3. Colonic irrigations
4. Colectomy (removal of the colon)
5. Recolonisation with lactobacilli (oral or rectal implants)
6. Specific high fibre diets
7. Improved blood flow to bowel
8. Allergy treatments (elimination and rotation diets)
9. Pancreatic support (enzyme supplementation)
10. Liver support

Detoxification with vitamin C

No discussion on detoxification would be complete or even meaningful without vitamin C — ascorbic acid. This very important nutrient is discussed in detail in the chapter on vitamin C and the bioflavonoids. Ascorbic acid has a number of possible actions and a number of definite actions as a detoxifying agent. First, and foremost, it is the prime free radical scavenger in the water soluble compartments of the body. Second, ascorbic acid is essential for the proper functioning of some of the detoxifying enzymes in the liver including glucuronidase and various hydroxylases. Third, ascorbic acid has been shown to prevent conversion of harmless chemicals into carcinogenic substances, for example the conversion of nitrites to nitrosamines in the gut. Ascorbic acid also acts as a reducing agent to keep other substances such as vitamin E, glutathione peroxidase, catalase and other enzymes active and functioning normally.

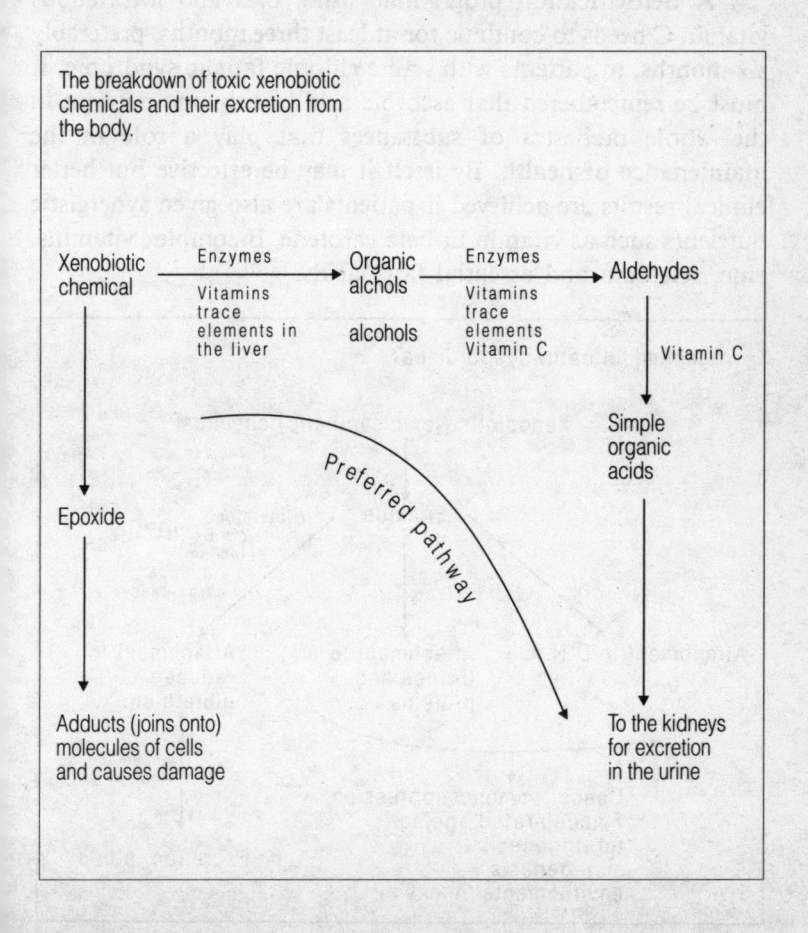

```
The breakdown of toxic xenobiotic
chemicals and their excretion from
the body.

Xenobiotic  --Enzymes-->  Organic  --Enzymes-->  Aldehydes
chemical    Vitamins      alchols  Vitamins
            trace                  trace
            elements in  alcohols  elements
            the liver              Vitamin C    |
                                                | Vitamin C
                                                v
                                                Simple
                                                organic
                                                acids
   |
   v                    Preferred pathway
Epoxide    ─────────────────────────────────>
   |                                            To the kidneys
   v                                            for excretion
Adducts (joins onto)                            in the urine
molecules of cells
and causes damage
```

There have been many studies to show that ascorbic acid can reduce the toxicity of inorganic poisons such as the heavy metals, mercury, arsenic, lead, chromium and gold and thousands of studies have shown that it can protect against organic poisons including drugs, anaesthetics, benzene, bacterial toxins and even snake bite and spider bite. Many more studies are needed on the effect of vitamin C in the chronic fatigue syndrome. However, at this point it can be shown that vitamin C is of definite benefit in the detoxification process when toxins, heavy metals, organic poisons, and by-products of bowel metabolism can be implicated in the cause of symptoms.

A detoxification programme using oral and intravenous vitamin C needs to continue for at least three months, preferably six months, in patients with severe chronic fatigue syndrome. It must be remembered that ascorbic acid is only one nutrient in the whole orchestra of substances that play a role in the maintenance of health. By itself it may be effective but better clinical results are achieved if patients are also given synergistic nutrients such as vitamin E, beta carotene, B-complex vitamins, zinc, selenium and essential fatty acids.

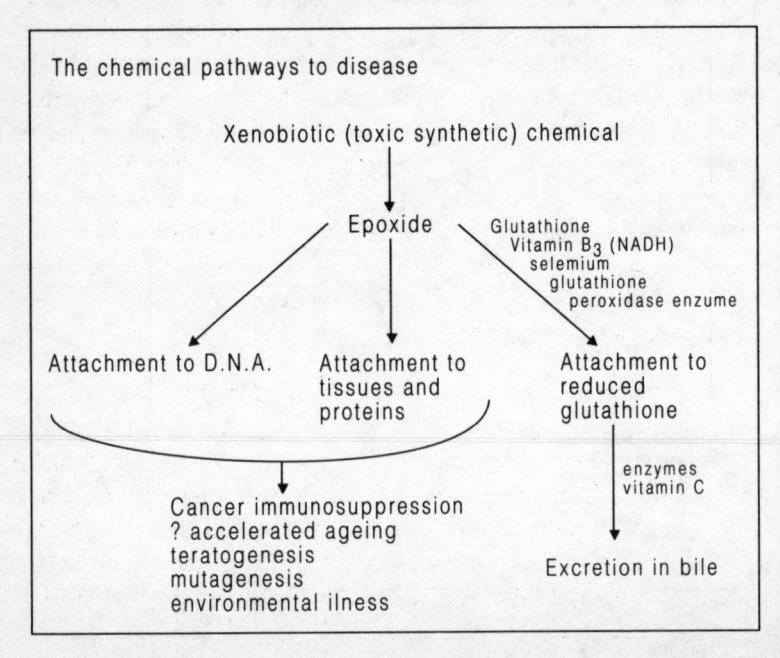

The chemical pathways to disease

Xenobiotic (toxic synthetic) chemical
↓
Epoxide

Glutathione
Vitamin B_3 (NADH)
selemium
glutathione
peroxidase enzume

- Attachment to D.N.A.
- Attachment to tissues and proteins
- Attachment to reduced glutathione

Cancer immunosuppression
? accelerated ageing
teratogenesis
mutagenesis
environmental ilness

↓ enzymes vitamin C

Excretion in bile

Chelation therapy

The word chelate is derived from the Greek word chele which refers to the claw of the crab. The word itself implies a firm pincher like action or binding effect. In biological terms, chelation is the binding of a metal to an organic or inorganic molecule. In chelation therapy we talk about the binding of a chelating substance to heavy metals such as lead, zinc, mercury, cadmium etc.

Chelation therapy involves the administration of a chelating substance, called EDTA or Ethylenediaminetetraacet acid, usually by an intravenous infusion. It is not routinely used in orthodox medicine except for patients with heavy metal poisonings. In the chronic fatigue syndrome it can be demonstrated by full hair analysis that as many as 30% of patients have high levels of heavy metals in their system. The hair analysis is the most accurate method of measuring these heavy metals and an assessment of the total toxic load of heavy metals can be obtained from this test. If the levels are high, and there has been no response to any other form of therapy, chelation should be seriously considered. In the right hands, the use of intravenous EDTA, 2 to 3grams in 500mls of intravenous fluid daily, is extremely safe. Providing the patient has good kidney function, and kidney function is monitored closely, the removal of heavy metals by this method can be extremely rewarding. Vitamins C, B-complex and minerals are given simultaneously. Between three and twenty chelation treatments administered on a daily basis are generally recommended. Some patients may feel an improvement after only three or four chelations. In this group of patients it is recommended that a total of between six and ten treatments are given.

Georgio's lead overload

> Two years ago Georgio, a young foundry worker, was divorced. According to his GP, Georgio had a mild nervous breakdown following the stress of the separation from his family. The 'breakdown' lasted longer than expected and after six months Georgio decided to seek help. Although an improved diet and vitamin supplements prescribed to him by a natural therapist helped, he continued to suffer periods of incapacitating fatigue.

> After discovering that his body's lead levels were extremely high, Georgio underwent intravenous chelation therapy to remove the lead. Before he had completed the course of 20 treatments, his health had remarkably improved, he was working as a building supervisor and he had developed a new and happy relationship.
>
> The suspected source of Georgio's poisoning was the lead contaminated air in the foundry where he previously worked, compounded by the lead from car fuels in the city air.

It is pointless giving chelation therapy if the source of heavy metal intoxification persists. Nothing can be done about the leaching out of lead from the bones into the bloodstream during chelation therapy. However, something can be done about other sources of lead especially if patients live near busy highways where the air is polluted from motor car exhausts.

Similarly, the patient with high levels of mercury will only benefit temporarily from chelation therapy if nothing is done about their mercury-silver amalgam dental fillings. Careful removal of dental amalgam fillings by a properly trained dentist using special dams and replacement with modern resins is recommended if mercury levels are high or mercury sensitivity can be demonstrated.

Other less significant heavy metals in respect to the chronic fatigue syndrome are cadmium, arsenic and aluminium. However, the presence of these toxic metals even in small amounts can add significantly to the total toxic heavy metal load.

Another very important aspect of chelation therapy in the chronic fatigue syndrome is the effect of EDTA on the mitochondria in muscle cells. Mitochondria are very small membrane bound organelles present in every cell of the body. They are basically the power houses of the cells and are responsible for transforming the energy in the foods we eat (glucose) into high energy phosphate bonds of a chemical called ATP. Estimations are that there are from between 200 and 2,000 mitochondria occur in every single cell. Within each mitochondria are as many as 10,000 complete sets of enzymes responsible for the oxidation processes which produce water, carbon dioxide and energy from our food fuels. Every living function and activity of the cell is dependent upon these mitochondria to release energy from food and transform that energy into a means by which the cell can use it. These energies may be present in the form of chemical energies, electrical energies (for example the nervous system) and transporting energies. ATP molecules produced by the mitochondria are the source of what is known as high energy phosphate bonds for the energy requiring activities of the cells. EDTA has been shown to actually restore normal functioning of damaged mitochondria either partially or completely in damaged calf muscle cells. This is extremely interesting when considering the cardinal symptom in the chronic fatigue syndrome is severe muscle fatigue. Here we are considering the basic molecular units involved in the production of energy, that is mitochondria and ATP. The function of these units can be improved by the use of a chelating agent such as EDTA.

Ascorbic acid (vitamin C) has been demonstrated to also have moderate chelating activity and at the molecular level one may postulate that this is where it acts. In a few patients with extremely severe chronic fatigue syndrome, a synergistic effect between the use of ascorbic acid and EDTA together has been observed.

Although EDTA chelation therapy treatment is not a recognised form of medical treatment in this country for the chronic fatigue syndrome, it is being used quite extensively in America and Europe for many conditions, including syndromes associated with fatigue. EDTA is a drug and when used in skilled hands, it is very safe. Providing the patient has good kidney function and is monitored appropriately during treatment, no untoward side effects should occur. It is not to be regarded as a first line of treatment and it should be reserved for those patients with severe chronic fatigue syndrome who have not, or only partially, responded to the other therapies described in this book.

The integrity of the bowel

In the study of physiology in medical schools and science faculties it was taught that the large molecules in foods were broken down into their individual units by the process of digestion. These units were than absorbed across the membrane of the bowel into the body circulation. These large molecules include proteins, polysaccharides, nucleic acids, glycoproteins, and they are made up of amino acids, simple sugars such as glucose and fructose and other simple compounds.

However, it is now known that these large molecules are not necessarily broken down completely and that they can pass across the bowel membrane barrier into the circulation as whole molecules. Appreciable quantities of proteins, nucleic acids, polypeptides and glycoproteins can actually penetrate the normally protective intestinal barrier to enter the bloodstream and eventually evoke an immunological reaction. This may be the mechanism by which foods cause allergies and sensitivities in some patients.

In the chronic fatigue syndrome, there are higher levels of antibodies of the IgE and IgG4 classes against food antigens than there is in the normal population. In patients suffering from the chronic fatigue syndrome, severe lethargy, tiredness and fatigue, associated with muscular aches and pains or abdominal symptoms, occurring within 30 minutes of eating is highly suggestive of a food or chemical sensitivity reaction.

Another important aspect of the permeability of the intestine to substances is that of the absorption of bacterial proteins, endotoxins, bacterial toxins and breakdown products of poorly digested food in the large intestine. This chemical cocktail in the large intestine has the potential to cause immune reactions, hormonal actions, toxic effects and effects on the body's pain relieving chemicals called endorphins. Interestingly, a breakdown product of some bacteria called muramyl dipeptide has been shown to enhance slow wave sleep. This dipeptide, produced in the bowel, has a number of other effects. These include the prevention of the effects of morphine withdrawal, elevation of the body temperature, interference with opiate receptors and it enhances the activity of some of the immune systems own chemicals (interleukin). It may be postulated that this dipeptide, or a similar substance, actually plays a role in the causes of the chronic fatigue syndrome. In some patients with CFS where bowel toxicity problems can be demonstrated, the sterilization of the bowel using natural or synthetic antibiotics and the replacement of the flora with lactobacillus acidophilus and bifidobacteria can result in dramatic improvement in their condition. More research should be done in this area to define the actual mechanisms.

There is a wide variety of microorganisms in the bowel. Over four hundred species of bacteria and fungi have been isolated from the bowel; in fact, the faeces consist of approximately 10 billion bacterial cells per gram of weight. These microorganisms are alive and metabolically active. They can produce 'allergies' and they secrete chemicals that may be beneficial or harmful. The beneficial chemicals include antibiotic-like substances and immune modulating agents. Harmful chemicals include toxins to the liver, brain, nervous system, and hormone glands. Others have even been demonstrated to act as carcinogens and cancer-promoting factors.

Approximately 15% people with the chronic fatigue syndrome have moderate to severe sugar and/or alcohol cravings from time to time. These cravings usually correlate to the severity of the clinical illness. The test that is usually performed is a glucose tolerance test. This demonstrates whether a patient has diabetes (high blood sugar) or reactive hypoglycaemia (low blood sugar). Neither of these conditions are usual in the patient with the chronic fatigue syndrome. However, abnormal sugar handling is usually demonstrated in the glucose test that is suggestive of borderline diabetes and/or reactive hypoglycaemia. The interpretation of the extended (6 hour) glucose tolerance test should be left in the hands of experts such as doctors who specialise in nutritional and environmental medicine. The point of the discussion here on blood sugar control and the microorganisms present in the bowel is not widely appreciated both by the lay public and healthcare professionals.

Blood sugar control is determined by the diet and a number of hormones including insulin secreted by the pancreas and glucagon secreted by the liver. Insulin reduces the blood sugar level. It has been shown that some bacteria in the large intestine can produce insulin-like molecules which interfere with the body's normal insulin activity. If this insulin-like molecule disturbs blood glucose levels, then the delivery of glucose to the nerves, muscles and other tissues of the body is adversely affected. This may be one of the mechanisms by which the fatigue syndrome is produced but again more research work needs to be done in this area.

Other bacteria in the bowel can produce protein-like molecules that may stimulate the body to produce antibodies that can interfere with the normal functioning of the nervous system.

Still other bacteria may interfere with the normal functioning of the thyroid gland.

Without doubt, the health of the intestine and large bowel plays an important role in the health of the patient with the chronic fatigue syndrome — the extent of which is yet to be fully appreciated.

CHAPTER NINE

Mind Power

Relaxation

We all need to relax our mind and body at least once a day. In some societies it becomes almost a ritual to relax once, twice or more often throughout a busy working day. For example, some middle-eastern and eastern religions require their devotees to stop their day-to-day routine and bow to Mecca or pray to God frequently. Even the non-religious Yogis of the east suggest punctuating the day with periods of rest and relaxation.

Everyone, no matter what their age or occupation, needs to have rest. The daily cycles of life and living dictate that periods of rest and activity are normal and that they are in-built mechanisms in every living thing.

Remember, just a few minutes relaxation at the same time every day is probably worth more to you than all of the hustling and bustling of everyday life. Complete relaxation and rest from your daily routine will bring renewed vigour, energy and peace of mind to the rest of your busy day. Relaxation isn't harmful. Drug therapies often are.

The question is — how do we do it?

Relaxation is an art. It is one of the aspects of daily living that is not adequately taught in schools or to our children generally. As babies, we develop the art of relaxing and switching off. As we become exposed to more external pressures and stimuli, these detract from this natural process of 'shifting into neutral gear'.

One of the best definitions of relaxation is 'to rest and enjoy yourself'. This means to stop doing and thinking about your everyday cares and worries and to turn away from the routine external environment. The idea is to focus on your pleasant thoughts — whatever they may be. Focusing on a different and pleasant activity is another way.

At the beginning, this process requires a certain amount of training and discipline to actually be able to concentrate on past experiences which have been of immense pleasure or plan future similar experiences.

The ability to concentrate within yourself is a learned activity. It requires practice and patience. It is simple and easy. One of the most effective ways to achieve this centring ability is to concentrate on your breathing. There are many different techniques for learning how to breath for relaxation and meditation and the following is probably as good as any.

Breathing to relax

Remember the last time you were tense and upset about something? What happened to your breathing? With most people in situations of tension, stress and anxiety, their breathing becomes more rapid and shallow. This short, rapid breathing actually promotes more tension and anxiety.

The ancients discovered that the control of breathing can control other activities in the nervous system. By reducing the rate of breathing, that is, by increasing the depth and time between each breath, it has been shown that not only can the breathing be slowed down but the rest of the activity in the nervous system also slows. This results in a feeling of relaxation. Thus, it can be seen that breathing rhythms and cycles are linked with the state of activity of the brain and mind. When you are calm, you breathe slowly and regularly. But when you are tense and anxious, you breathe quickly and shallowly. By controlling the breathing, and therefore the brain and mind, this tension can be switched off.

One of the simplest, most effective ways of controlling breathing is the following exercise. Sit on the floor with your legs crossed and your back straight. Concentrate on breathing out slowly through your nose. As you breathe, imagine a feather being held a few inches away from your nostrils.

Concentrate on breathing in and breathing out slowly through the nose so that the imagined feather hardly moves. The slower and the deeper you can make the breaths, the better. At the beginning, this may seem difficult, but concentrate on it. Count the number of seconds it takes to inhale and exhale each time. When you start these exercises, you may only be able to breathe in to the count of five seconds and out to the count of five seconds. Practise increasing the number to ten seconds on inhalation and ten seconds on exhalation.

When you have achieved this slow, rhythmical breathing, you can increase the counts up to twenty seconds. Count slowly and quietly to yourself. In time, you will be able to make this practice a routine with which you can punctuate your day. You may find that doing it once or twice a day is sufficient to keep you relaxed. You may even find that by performing these controlled breathing exercises four to six times during the day, you feel better, have more energy, work more efficiently and have greater control and intuition.

Once you have learned to control your breathing like this, a short period of controlled breathing exercises before retiring is an ideal way of slowing down your breathing rhythms and activity in the brain.

Don't worry about any other fancy techniques of breathing, because once you have mastered this technique, you are well on the way to self-control and relaxation. Remember, the feather in front of the nose. It should still be there and slightly quivering towards the nose on inhalation with a very gentle movement away from the nose on exhalation.

This is how slow, deliberate and gentle the breathing should be. This is what life should be. With slow, gentle, rhythmic, controlled breathing, all mind and body activities follow naturally.

Controlled breathing

- Practise three times a day
- Practise when feeling early stress
- Remember: longer breaths, slower breaths, deeper breaths
- Practise before bed

Meditation

Meditation is probably the single most powerful therapy in the management of any disease. It has been practised for centuries in eastern countries to maintain health and well-being and to aid in recovery from illness. Its psychological effects include relief from tension and anxiety, and a feeling of inner calmness. The physical effects include the relief of pain and physical discomfort, the reduction of metabolic activity, the activation of the immune system and the normalisation of many physiological activities including heart rate, blood pressure and respiration.

Meditation creates a definite mental harmony and emotional balance in people who practise it. Coinciding with this improved mental harmony is the improvement in overall wellness, increased energy and the ability to sleep better.

'When the apple is ripe it will drop from the tree of its own weight'.

This eastern proverb beautifully sums up the meaning of meditation. The meditative process acts as a catalyst to organise the body's chemistry into a whole. The mind has profound influences on our degree of health. Even in sickness it can play a role either by improving the degree of wellness or worsening the degree of illness.

Not only do thoughts and emotions influence our behaviour, but these very thoughts and emotions can play a direct role in influencing all of the body's subtle physical and chemical actions and reactions.

The time-honoured method of meditation has recently become very popular in the management of many illnesses, including cancer, AIDS, psychosomatic disorders, pain and high blood pressure. Meditation has been scientifically validated as a method of improving physical and psychological functioning.

A spin-off of all this improvement of course is more energy during the day and better sleep at night.

The act of meditation generates positive behaviour and attitudes without effort or cost. With a modest investment of time, meditation can take you to a higher plane of well-being and a totally different perspective on your existence.

Meditation is the foundation for optimum health. It is not a religion but a way of life. Meditation is concentration within. It is effortless. It is just as if you are falling down a well within yourself. Others have described it as a 'diving within'.

Meditation is simply the process of being able to effortlessly let go of everything while concentrating on one thought, one word or one idea. In fact, simply sitting and knitting can be regarded as a form of meditation.

By passively sitting in a chair in a slightly uncomfortable position with your eyes closed for twenty minutes twice a day, you can eventually achieve a state of relaxation or meditation. The mind is allowed to wander and invading thoughts are allowed to pass through consciousness. Eventually the concentration within starts to dominate. This may take days, weeks, even months, depending upon the individual. All thoughts are eventually blocked out using this process.

By achieving the ability to switch off in such a way, this well-practised habit of meditation can be applied in the evening before bedtime. By allowing the mind to calm itself, sleep naturally follows. The intellect is gradually phased out. It is not necessary to think during the meditative process. No conscious effort is required and increased feelings of inner peace, deep relaxation and serenity usually develop. Eventually, even the feelings of inner peace fade away to be replaced by a state of selflessness. This gently progresses into a deep feeling of unity, or oneness, with the entire self and your surroundings.

When you are at peace with yourself, not only do you feel better within but you can notice improvements in your relationships.

The 'meditation habit' takes time. It cannot be developed overnight or even within days or weeks. A slow transition occurs in yourself after you have practised meditation for several months. This change is slow but sure. On a day-to-day basis, changes are usually not very noticeable. However, over several weeks blending into months, you will find tremendous changes.

Meditation proceeds at its own speed and reaches its goal in its own time. The whole process should be allowed to flow naturally and slowly.

Meditation can help a large number of disease states which may, or may not, be associated with insomnia. It has helped thousands of cancer patients and millions of patients with immune disorders and allergies world-wide.

People who meditate say that they can cope better with the realities of life. They become more resilient to external, irritating factors and they feel more together 'within' themselves. They have more energy, feel more spontaneous and less tense. It appears that their whole coping and adaptive mechanism improves. Overall, people become more cheerful and optimistic and find that they can more easily accept their day-to-day problems. However, there is a cost — time and self-discipline.

It is equally important for a person who is well as it is for someone suffering from the chronic fatigue syndrome or some other severe disease to approach meditation with a deep degree of sincerity, openness and a genuine desire to learn about themselves. In other words, it is a feeling of needing and wanting to reach out for something deeper and more meaningful.

Some people who have undertaken meditation have found that previous experiences can be relived extremely vividly. They note that their reactions to these experiences in the past may have been inappropriate and immature. By reliving these experiences and by changing their responses purposefully, a sense of greater self-esteem and personal growth results.

Simple, natural, effective

Meditation is a simple therapy. It can be practised at any time. It is a safe and sure method which can be used by all, including children. Meditation is not prayer and it is not a religion. It is not self-hypnosis but it does resemble such a state of mind. It is also not a form of magic or a secret formula derived from ancient mystics. The state of meditation is certainly not learning the ability to develop alpha brain waves or any other fancy scientific explanation.

Meditation is a natural process. Observe your pet dog or cat lying in front of a warm fire. They are not always asleep when their eyes are closed. In fact, your pet is probably meditating on the soft warmth of the fire and the homely sound of voices.

Meditation may be as simple as sitting knitting, listening to music with the eyes closed or, more seriously, the purposeful sitting in the lotus position with eyes closed concentrating on a word or thought. The lotus position is the classical yogic sitting position in which the legs are crossed and the feet are brought up to rest on the tops of the thighs.

Meditation is not a form of psychotherapy, although many people find it psychologically helpful. Meditation is simply a state of being and knowing within. The practised meditator will discover what this eventually means. The key word is practice.

Practising effective meditation

The successful practice of meditation requires a little time and self-discipline. With this investment you will find that your life can be dramatically changed. Not only will fatigue, insomnia, minor aches and pains, frustrations, anxieties, tensions and problems seem much better but the risk of developing serious illness is greatly reduced, including the reduced likelihood of a recurrence of the chronic fatigue syndrome once it is controlled.

But the determination to meditate must come from within yourself. For someone suffering from chronic fatigue and all of its associated symptoms, this is often quite difficult at the beginning. The discipline needed to spend half-an-hour twice a day on meditative practice must come from a genuine desire for self-improvement. The urge to fall asleep should be resisted.

Two half-hour daily sessions are recommended for a reasonably healthy individual. Some very sick patients who are benefiting from diet and meditation spend two or more hours a day meditating and claim great improvement. Their secret is self-discipline and if you are willing to apply it, there is no reason why you cannot beat your fatigue and the symptoms that go along with it.

Select a quiet room and use the same place each time for your meditation. The bedroom is ideal. Lock the door and either take the telephone off the hook or turn the bell down. Make sure that you are not distracted by anyone or anything, including distracting thoughts.

The room must be very, very quiet. It is important to select the same time every day to meditate. That is, it is very important to develop a good meditation habit. Choose a chair which isn't too comfortable. A comfortable chair will enable you to fall asleep. The best chair is one in which you're sitting without back support.

The best time to meditate is early in the morning and late in the afternoon. You must meditate twice a day. Each time you meditate, you should take twenty to thirty minutes — therefore you will be meditating for forty to sixty minutes daily to start with.

When you do become more familiar with the routine, you will naturally increase your meditation time if and when required. It is possible to meditate for six or more hours a day. This may be necessary for some very sick people. However, my recommendations are forty to sixty minutes daily for most people. Once the habit of meditation has been adopted and it is being practised effectively, a ten-minute session in the middle of the day can be quite relieving and invigorating.

You must carefully prepare yourself for each meditation session. Don't use alcohol or stimulants such as tea, coffee, tobacco, or other drugs before meditation. Obviously, it is not really a good idea to use these at any time! It is also important not to get excited or involved in an overstimulating session with friends or workmates.

It is better to meditate before a meal than after. Experienced meditators find that an empty stomach is more conducive to the true meditative process. If you need to go to the toilet, then do so. There is no point in meditating with a bowel or bladder that is wanting to empty itself. Be as comfortable as possible. Wear loose clothing but sufficient to keep you warm in the winter.

Sit perfectly quietly on the edge of your chosen chair, straighten the back and hold your head up. Attempt to emphasise the curves in your lower back as much as possible. Your hands should be placed on your lap close to the knees. At this stage, you are ready to allow your thoughts to flow freely, 'like a river', while concentrating on your breathing. The concentration on the breathing should be on definite, slow inhalations and exhalations. Imagine a feather in front of the nose just moving towards and away from your nose with each inhalation and exhalation.

A state of free thinking is the key to successful meditation. Don't worry about pleasant, or unpleasant, thoughts appearing. In time, your thoughts will change in a way that will help you to meditate more effectively. If you are in the habit of using affirmations repeat these over and over again at the beginning of each meditation session. In this way, your thoughts can be concentrated on to a few affirmative sentences.

Affirmations which are ideal to start with are: 'I have more energy'; 'I feel good about myself'; 'Every day, in every way, I'm getting better and better'; 'I'm relaxed and happy at all times.' Or you can, of course, make up your own.

Just relax and let it happen

Breathe very slowly inwardly and outwardly through your nose. It is possible to reduce the amount of breathing to two or three breaths or less in a minute. Don't force yourself at all. I repeat, the entire process is meant to be effortless.

It is easy, it is simple and it works. But, remember — twice a day in the same place for at least twenty to thirty minutes. Don't expect immediate results or rewards. These come in time. Make meditation a lifetime practice and many of your problems will be solved — and the others will seem less important.

Meditation and sleep

The effects of meditation are not conducive to immediate sleep, despite its calming and restful effects.

The effect of sleep and insomnia come as a result of the altered state of physiology of the body and mind. That is, if we can remain relaxed calm and peaceful during the day from our meditation sessions, then the fall of night comes with a feeling of peaceful fatigue and the desire for natural sleep.

Meditation and food

Excessive food can influence sleep and disturb our state of rest. It can also disturb our ability to meditate and focus on a particular thought. It is unwise to eat immediately before or after a meditation session because food itself can interrupt the delicate and subtle physiological changes which occur.

From this form of meditation, you will only gain what you are prepared to give. Once you have become an experienced meditator you will get more from the meditation than you actually put into it. Most people find that it usually takes from one to three months before they know if they are benefiting from the sessions. Again, this depends on the individual and the amount of time that is devoted to the discipline of the meditative exercise.

Awareness and energy improve

A change in your level of awareness is probably the first change which occurs in the first few months of meditation. Sometimes this occurs earlier and, within a period of days to weeks, meditation brings results. Also, by being able to relax and switch off the stresses and tension during the day, the stress-tension-fatigue cycle can be interrupted.

Meditation is a form of recharging your batteries. However, the increased level of relaxation and the reduction in anxiety levels are two of the more obvious changes which occur in the early phases of the meditative process.

It is important to realise that meditation is a total clearing of all thoughts and fears. Invading thoughts are allowed to enter and become a part of the mind for the process of meditation. However, attempts should always be made to clear these thoughts as soon as possible.

Repetition of affirmations is one way of switching off thoughts which may appear to be too intrusive. Of course, fears and guilts will arise, as will past experiences. These must also be dealt with in the same way. Not by blocking them off but by allowing them to flow freely. If they become persistent and over-invasive, then attempt to waylay them by using your affirmations. Allow thoughts to enter the mind and to pass through unhindered. This constant practice will allow you to gain control of your thoughts, actions and behaviour and, indirectly, it will result in you being able to control your symptoms.

Keep the mind as a form of register

You must attempt to treat the mind as a form of register. The register must be cleared at the beginning of each session. Alternatively, it can be thought of as a tape which can be magnetically cleared of all information at will. When the tape is replayed, nothing appears in it.

This is what is meant by the process of meditation. The mind should eventually be clear of all thoughts. In time, an experienced meditator can apply meditation anywhere — in a busy train, at work or on the top of a mountain. However, to start with it is desirable to meditate in a comfortable, quiet, familiar place. The bedroom is ideal. Don't worry if the whole process seems slow. It is! Things are still happening to you but at a pace at which your mind and body will allow. The important points to remember are regular practice and don't try too hard.

Cooking a small fish

The two most common mistakes are trying too hard — and not trying enough. Trying too hard happens when you try to concentrate too much or begin to intellectualise or become impatient and attempt to speed up the whole meditative process.

On the other hand, not trying enough occurs when you slip out of your routine of meditating twice a day. Don't let the sessions become superficial by allowing distractions to occur.

Also, insufficient attempts at meditation occur when you cut the session short or fall asleep. The Chinese describe this process of doing but not overdoing as like 'cooking a small fish - you must be careful not to overdo it.'

Without effort

The experience of meditation will take you into a realm of quiet and subdued expectancy in which you become open and receptive to everything.

This is an effortless process requiring time and self-discipline only. Experienced meditators become attuned to everything. But, they hear or see nothing at first and have no expectations of what is to occur before, or after the meditation. They are therefore really never disappointed.

Whatever happens to them is usually for the best. As far as you are concerned, the meditation process requires virtually no effort at all. However, the rewards of meditation come when you are ready. They come at their own speed, and in their own time, and they cannot be hurried.

CHAPTER TEN

An anti-fatigue management programme

Principles to remember

In the approach to any health problem three important principles must always be applied:
1. An accurate diagnosis.
2. The removal of the causes, aggravating factors and symptomatic treatment.
3. The optimisation of the health status and environment of the individual.

These factors are discussed in depth in this book. With most medical conditions, orthodox medicine performs extremely well on principle No. 1, moderately well on principle No. 2 but, to-date, has been unable to come to grips with the holistic methods required for the induction of health optimisation and environmental medicine.

Inherited weaknesses in immune function are well known and a number of diseases of the immune system are genetically acquired. For example, a disease called primary immunodeficiency or ataxia telangiectasia is determined by genetic factors. However, it is highly likely but not yet defined that other factors inherited by an individual in their genes may adversely affect expression of these genes in immune functioning.

To take a simple example of this, many people in the community can escape the common cold and influenza epidemics year after year and yet others are extremely susceptible to them and may contract more than one virus every winter. We may argue that those people who suffer from these infections more often than not are under more stress, don't eat well and perhaps abuse themselves with tobacco, alcohol and other drugs. However, this is not necessarily the case for in careful history taking it is often revealed that these individuals suffered from more frequent respiratory infections as infants and children. The pointer here is to a genetic weakness and perhaps other system malfunctioning. Although periconceptual nutritional factors may play a role in immune functioning in the offspring, it is beyond the scope of this book to discuss the importance of nutrition in the parents and even grandparents prior to conception. We know from scientific studies that if rats are deprived of zinc during pregnancy the offspring will show weaknesses in their immune system due to their mother's zinc deficiency state during pregnancy. These offspring will pass on this weakness to their offspring for another three or four generations down the line. This is despite adequate zinc nourishment of all those subsequent generations of rats. Whether this occurs in humans or not is debatable and very little evidence exists to support this concept. However, we know from clinical experience that some families are more susceptible to immune and infectious type disorders, including allergic diseases, than others. In clinical practice, it is also observed in these families that if diet is improved and simple nutrient supporting supplements like vitamin C, B-complex and zinc are provided, then the atopic or allergic state improves and may even disappear over a period of time.

Intertwining themselves within these basic principles of care are the holistic facets of health optimisation. These include a concentrated patient-centred approach to management which is comprehensive in extent and multifactorial in nature, encompassing orthodox and alternative complementary and natural healing methodologies. Holistic care does not exist in a stressful environment and emphasises non-toxic (but not exclusively) drug-free care. Psychological and spiritual factors may play a minor to major part in holism, depending upon the particular and individual circumstances.

Summary of treatment of fatigue

1. Most importantly, the patient and the doctor must recognise the syndrome and then eliminate the medical and psychiatric causes of fatigue e.g. anaemia, heart disease, depression, diabetes, cancer etc.
2. Investigate and treat food sensitivity and allergy.
3. Investigate and treat chemical sensitivity, or overload.
4. Investigate and treat environmental factors including inhalant allergies, electro-magnetic radiation factors and the 'sick building' syndrome.
5. Correct vitamin and mineral balances and deficiencies.
6. Correct any other nutrient imbalances or deficiencies including essential fatty acids, trace elements and amino acid therapy.
7. Diet with nutrient dense foods and food rotation.
8. Stimulate immune function, non-specific and specific immune stimulating agents, e.g. the herbs echinacea, glycyrrhiza, galium, and zinc and antioxidants.
9. Address any problems with infestations of parasites and candida, especially in the bowel.
10. Protect cells and tissues with antioxidant nutrients and compounds.
11. Utilise detoxification methods especially for the large bowel and liver.
12. Improve circulation of the blood and lymphatics.
13. Evaluate for mercury toxicity and sensitivity (include other heavy metals also).
14. Institute specific herbal therapies for symptomatic relief and specific organ nourishment.
15. Encourage appropriate physical exercise.
16. Provide oxygen therapies when indicated.
17. Insist on some form of positive thinking, mind control or meditation with affirmations.
18. Evaluate the worthiness of homeopathic remedies and acupuncture if appropriate.

19. Encourage as much social interaction as possible.
20. Do not use prescription drugs unless they are absolutely necessary eg. pain killers, tranquillisers or anti-depressants.

As stress, poor diet and chemicals are the main ingredients in the production of ill health, their correction is vital for a full recovery. Factors in correcting them, in order of importance are:
1. Strict adherence to diet
2. A reduction in the level of stress, plus adequate rest and relaxation
3. Appropriately prescribed nutritional supplements
4. Adequate gentle exercise such as yoga

The diet entails the strict avoidance of:
■ Sugar rich foods such as confectionery, soft drinks, glucose, honey, malt, cane sugar containing foods, sweet biscuits, cakes, deserts, golden syrup, molasses, dried fruits, sweet dried fruits, raisins, dates, figs, sultanas etc. Fruit juices should be diluted 50% with mineral water or preferably purified water with a maximum of two glasses of diluted juice per day. ■ White flour products and refined starchy foods such as white bread, biscuits, pasta, pastries, pies, sauces, gravies and canned and bottled foods which may contain white flour as a filling or bulking agent. ■ Coffee and conventional tea. These are unnecessary stimulants which have been shown to increase levels of anxiety thus interfering with any attempts to reduce stress in the unwell person. Coffee has also been proven to raise the levels of cholesterol in the blood. Both are associated with high rates of certain cancers. Preferably drink 'purified' tap water and herbal teas. For information concerning effective water purifiers (not filters), contact the Allergy Aid Centre in your capital city. ■ All alcoholic beverages ■ All tobacco products, cigarette smoke, drugs (unless medically prescribed), environmental pollutants including chemicals used at work and in the home and food additives. ■ The strict avoidance of all foods and chemicals that are causing sensitivity reactions shown by blood tests, skin tests, sublingual challenges or food provocations.

Protein rich snacks

Frequent snacks of protein-rich foods in between meals are often helpful in times of stress and provided the snacks are kept small, weight should remain stable. This is a form of 'grazing' and it is particularly helpful in people who have problems with digestion and symptoms in the abdomen. Instead of consuming three large meals a day, 6 to 8 small snacks are eaten. These snacks should consist of as many different foods as possible, to avoid repetition and to supply a wide range of nutrients. Protein rich snacks could include the following (vegetarians select only the non-animal protein sources):

- Unsalted nuts e.g. hazel, almonds, cashews
- Seeds e.g. sunflower, pumpkin — both are more easily digested if they are softened by soaking in water for a couple of hours before eating.
- Legumes and pulses including peas, beans, unsalted peanut butter, lentils etc.
- Thick pea soup
- Hard-boiled free-range eggs
- Thick lentil soup
- Fish
- Veal
- Steak
- Poultry
- Lamb's fry
- Bean curd (tofu), chick pea dip (hommus)

Meals generally

Meals should generally contain a substantial protein component until the symptoms of stress have eased. Lean meat, grilled fish and lamb's fry are all beneficial. Alternatively, dishes made from vegetable proteins such as beans, bean curd, lentils, chick-peas, sesame and sunflower seeds and pumpkin seeds are ideal.

Free-range eggs and yoghurt are also good sources of protein but it must be stressed that if allergies are suspected, then avoidance of these foods may be necessary.

Plenty of fresh organically grown fruits and vegetables should be included and at least one third of the vegetables should be eaten raw. Lightly steam or quickly stir fry the remaining vegetables. Always avoid hidden sugars in meals and especially desserts and processed foods e.g. canned fruits, baked beans, breakfast cereals.

Dietary considerations

Although a significant proportion of people with CFS appear to benefit from the manipulation of their diet and the removal of foods to which they are sensitive, the nutritional approach is grossly incomplete if the elimination of a number of foods is the only management. It is simplistic and most unscientific.

Probably more important in this group of patients, many of whom have been shown to be suffering from multiple nutritional deficiencies, is the assessment of macro- and micro-nutrient balance. Deficiencies of zinc for example in this population group are extremely frequent. The assessment of zinc status must be correctly performed. To simply rely on a better diet to correct these zinc deficiencies is absolutely futile. In fact, by simply placing a patient on an elimination diet with or without rotation of foods is tantamount to negligence with regard to their specific nutritional needs. Aggravation of these deficiencies is highly possible on elimination diets. Arguably, the removal of foods causing sensitivities results in the enhanced absorbtion rate of nutrients from the small intestine. However, this does not ensure the satisfactory correction of nutrient deficiencies or imbalances.

Some medical researchers still believe that patients may recover from CFS spontaneously without any active treatment at all. However, it has been the experience of the practitioners in the nutritional and environmental medicine movement that most patients who have been documented by medical researchers as having a spontaneous recovery have in actual fact recovered as a consequence of so-called alternative or complementary medicine approaches. Indeed, it is unfortunate that medical researchers actually ignore the benefits obtained by CFS patients from modalities of treatment with which they are not familiar.

Common myths about nutrition

1. A well-balanced diet supplies all of the nutrients in sufficient quantities that we need for optimal health.
2. Processed foods contain nutrients sufficient for optimal health and disease prevention.

3. Our food supply contains safe levels of agricultural chemicals e.g. herbicide and pesticide residues.
4. If we suspect a nutritional deficiency then all we have to do is increase the quantity of food we eat to correct it.
5. Organic fruits and vegetables are safe to eat.
6. Chlorine and fluoride in the water are harmless in the doses that are added.
7. Vegetarianism is best for everybody.
8. Sugar is a natural part of a balanced diet.
9. Processing of food does very little harm, e.g. storing, packaging, freezing, colouring, processing, flavouring, gassing and irradiating it.
10. The selection of a variety of foods from the five major food groups is good nutrition for everyone. (This ignores the fact that over 10% of the Australian population have food sensitivities.)
11. Food allergies and food sensitivities are rare and affect less than 5% of the population.
12. Nutritional deficiencies are uncommon in modern western societies.
13. Fast take-away foods are an acceptable part of a balanced nutritional programme.
14. Alcohol is safe if consumed in small quantities.
15. Biological individuality is not important if a wide variety of foods are consumed.
16. The human body has evolved mechanisms that will allow it to detoxify the 60,000 chemicals it is exposed to in the environment.
17. Foods do not influence behaviour, learning or the emotions.
18. Dietary manipulation and therapeutic nutrition do not influence diseases that have a genetic component, e.g. cancer, diabetes, arthritis, cardiovascular disease.
19. Everybody's metabolism is basically the same and the concept of 'metabolic types' is a fallacy.
20. Fasting and juice diets are harmful.
21. Doctors and dietitians know enough about nutrition to provide the best advice.
22. The government has good control on the quality of our food supply.
23. Ice-cream and soft-drinks are good foods (according to some Australian dieticians).

24. Increasing vitamin intake does not improve health and generally increases the risk of harmful side effects. **Note** — vitamins are far safer than drugs — 20% of hospital beds are occupied by patients suffering from the side effects of medically prescribed drugs. There has only been rare instances of patients hospitalised from an overdose of a vitamins and the effects are totally reversible.
25. Australians do not consume an excessive quantity of junk food.
26. Foods do not have therapeutic properties e.g. they don't improve diseases such as the chronic fatigue syndrome, arthritis, heart disease, cancer, diabetes.
27. The mainline print and electronic media give unbiased information on diet and nutrition.
28. The only benefits derived from nutritional supplementation are due to the placebo effect and are based on anecdotal reports without hard scientific data.

Timing of meals

Body rhythms are becoming an important part of the study of biology and disease. There is good evidence to show that the normal body rhythms of people with the chronic fatigue syndrome are disturbed.

Daily, monthly and seasonal rhythms have been discovered. Biochemical changes occurring during the daily rhythms are a direct result of the interaction between inherent biotimes and biorhythms, the time of feeding and probably the type of foods eaten. Meal timing can affect body weight, hormone levels, blood pressure, mental alertness, body temperature, cell division and many other bodily functions.

Modern science is only just coming to terms with these cycles that ancient Chinese and Indian healers used in clinical practice for centuries. Our eating patterns are dictated by food supply, satiety, hunger, social habits, work pressures and convenience.

The consideration of meal timing has important implications concerning the body's ability to obtain optimum energy from the food consumed. For example, fats are utilised preferentially in the evening. The timing of the intake of foods that contain the precursors to stimulate neurotransmitter production, for example glycine, tryptophan and tyrosine, is particularly important in patients suffering from neuropsychiatric problems and depression. Neurotransmitter functions exhibit a spectrum of rhythms and these are reflected in hormonal changes. Alterations in the rhythms of the production of the hormones cortisol, melatonin and some hormones from the pituitary gland may be the harbingers for the risk of the development of depression, high blood pressure and even cancer.

Intervention by dietary means to correct these disturbances may turn out to be one or the most effective methods of preventing and treating these diseases.

In more than 90% of patients studied with the chronic fatigue syndrome, disturbances in both sleeping and eating patterns have been found. The two most common findings in these patients have been the missing of meals, especially breakfast, and the bingeing on or craving for refined carbohydrates, especially sugar.

From the perspective of what to eat and when, the most effective single piece of advice is to eat breakfast every day and this most important meal should contain good quality protein. A small piece of grilled, de-fatted red meat is ideal in the short term. Other protein rich foods are listed in this chapter.

Nutritional supplements — vitamins, minerals and antioxidants

The use of nutritional supplements is the single most effective treatment in the management of the chronic fatigue syndrome and its future prevention.

The following protocol is **essential** for all patients with CFS:
1. Vitamin C with bioflavonoids & quercetin — 1000mg three times a day.
2. High potency B-complex containing the exact concentrations of the following:
   Vitamin B1 — 50mg.   Nicotinic acid — 10mg.
   Vitamin B2 — 20mg.   Vitamin B3 — 200mg.

AN ANTI-FATIGUE MANAGEMENT PROGRAMME

     Vitamin B5 — 100mg.   Skullcap — 100mg.
     Vitamin B6 — 50mg.   Valerian — 100mg.
     Vitamin B12 — 100mcg. Glutamine — 50mg.
     Beta carotene — 3mg.   Lysine — 10mg.
     Vitamin E — 20mg.   Choline — 50mg.
     Biotin — 20mcg.   Inositol — 20mg.
     Folic acid — 150mcg.   Minerals
     Lithium — 140mcg.   Betaine HCl — 10mg.

     1/2 — 1-2 tablets three times a day.

3. Antioxidant formula with selenium (50mcg. selenium per tab.) 1 tablet three times a day.
4. Water soluble 'natural' vitamin E 250 units per capsule 1 capsule three times a day.
5. Halibut or cod liver oil capsules 2 capsules daily.
6. High potency GLA evening primrose oil capsules 2 capsules three times a day.
7. Multi-minerals containing calcium, magnesium, chromium, copper, iodine, iron, manganese, molybdenum, potassium 1 tablet three times a day.
8. Lactobacillus and bifidobacteria powder (mixed) 1 teaspoon in water three times a day before meals for one week, then once a day.
9. Zinc with manganese, cone flower and sarsaparilla (with 30mgm of elemental zinc) 1 tablet three times a day.
10. Injections:
    a) Daily injections of intravenous vitamin C, 15-30 grams or more depending on the clinical response for two weeks, reducing to twice weekly injections for one month and then weekly to fortnightly injections.
    b) Weekly or twice weekly injections of high potency B vitamins containing the following vitamins in exact proportions:
    Vitamin B1 — 250mgm.
    Vitamin B6 — 100mgm.
    Vitamin B12 — 1000mcg.
    Folic acid — 15mgm.

The following may be added to the above when indicated:
1. Liver nutrients for people with symptoms pertaining to the liver and gastrointestinal tract such as nausea, abdominal discomfort, flatulence, constipation etc. (dandelion, barberry, slippery elm, golden seal, greater celandine, boldo, choline, inositol, methionine, peppermint oil — these can be obtained in a single tablet.)
2. Bowel cleansing nutrients for severe constipation and toxic problems (psyllium, rhubarb, gentian, cascara).
3. Shitake and reishi mushrooms in powder form 1 teaspoon per day are especially useful in people who have been shown to have immune suppression or who suffer from recurrent infections. They are used extensively in the east and in Japanese medicine.
4. Herbal remedies for the nervous and immune systems include lomatium, astragalus, liquorice, phytolacca, baptisia, echinacea, panax ginseng, Siberian ginseng and mistletoe which is often given also by injection.
5. Biotin 300mcg per day will assist those with confirmed candida sensitivity as will the drugs Nystatin (500,000i.u. 4 times a day) or Ketoconazole 200 to 400mg. per day under medical supervision.
6. Garlic extracts are useful in heavy metal and bowel toxicities.
7. Selenium in medically monitored doses of 200 to 1000mcg per day are of benefit to patients with proven chemical sensitivities and mercury sensitivity/toxicity syndrome.
8. Total dental amalgam clearance in the resistant patient with high levels of toxic heavy metals in the hair analysis or mercury sensitivity. These people may also require intravenous chelation therapy to remove a substantial burden of heavy metals in their tissues.
9. Oxygen therapies including the use of intravenous and oral hydrogen peroxide and ozone have been reported to be of benefit in some patients, but these are not generally recommended unless under strict medical supervision including the monitoring of the patient's antioxidant status which may be compromised by oxidation processes.
10. Specific homoeopathic remedies carefully prescribed by an experienced homoeopath may bring about dramatic benefit,

but the above mentioned nutritional protocol improves the chances of successful homoeopathic treatments.
11. Glutamine 400 to 800mgm. three times a day before meals has been of benefit to people with symptoms of severe 'brain fag'. It is an important chemical for brain functioning and, being an amino acid found in foods, can be regarded as safe to take. However, it is recommended that glutamine be taken with vitamin C and the high potency B-complex mentioned above for best results.

Avoidance of chemicals

Although it is virtually impossible to avoid the multitude of chemical pollutants present in the air we breathe, the water we drink and the foods we eat, it is possible to reduce the 'total chemical load' on our bodies. The avoidance of deliberate and direct contact with garden and household chemicals is relatively simple. Cosmetics and perfumes are also major sources of chemical contamination. Highly polluted air in cities and industrial areas cause ear, nose, throat and lung problems for many. In farming areas, pesticide sprays can cause severe physical and psychological illnesses. In fact, virtually any symptom or disease can be caused or aggravated by synthetic or naturally occurring chemicals. Dr Richard Mackarness' book *Chemical Victims* has an appendix showing how to avoid excess chemical exposure.

Important affirmations

As a psychological aid and effective behavioural tool, the following series of affirmations should be repeated as many times as necessary during the day and last thing at night to achieve a more positive attitude of mind:
- Every day in every way I'm getting better and better and better.
- Negative thoughts do not influence me — I am always positive.
- I am always relaxed and happy.
- My energy levels are increasing.
- I am totally confident in all situations.

- I am under my own control — I am in control.

The principles of natural good health

1. Health is the normal condition of the body and under natural conditions it should continue from birth to death.
2. Health is that condition of the body when all of its functions perform harmoniously and it is maintained by living in accordance with nature.
3. The health of an organism is governed by eating habits, proper exercise, abundant sunshine, fresh air, pure water, rest, a positive mental attitude and the avoidance of all habits which devitalise the system and disturb the balance of bodily functions.
4. Disease is basically the reaction of the body to a departure from some of the conditions necessary for good health.
5. Health can be regained and maintained by living in harmony with nature and allowing the natural healing powers of the body to restore health.
6. Drugs, radiation and other similar treatments interfere with the bodies restorative power and so, while suppressing symptoms, retard the restoration of health. They are necessary for intervention for acute severe and life-threatening illnesses when there are no alternatives.
7. The same factors which are necessary to maintain health are also the basis for the control of disease conditions if they arise.
8. Incorrect eating habits, stress and chemical pollution are the principal causative factors in most of the health problems of civilised life.
9. The natural and most beneficial way to alleviate acute disease is through fasting — that is, complete abstention from both solid and liquid foods, consuming only pure water. Alternatively, diluted vegetable juices may be consumed, for example carrot or celery.
10. Chronic disease is the intensification of acute disease. It becomes manifest when the self-healing powers of the body are overtaxed.

Heat therapies

The history of heat therapies dates back to the ancient Chinese physicians who believed that certain body types responded to either heat or cold depending on the illness. The great classical Greek physician Parmenides told his followers two thousand years ago — 'Give me a chance to create a fever and I will cure any disease'. Fever, that is a raised temperature due to an increase in body heat, is one of the greatest defence mechanisms. It creates an increase in the metabolic rate as a consequence of infection. The result of this high temperature actually inhibits the growth of infecting viruses, bacteria and fungi. In fact, before the advent of penicillin and other wonder antibiotics, one of the treatments for syphilis and other infectious diseases, was the production of fever. The use of heat treatments, saunas and fever therapy in the health clinics of Europe is not restricted to the treatment of infectious diseases. It is also used in the management of other serious degenerative disorders including arthritis, diabetes, leukaemia and cancer. The Arapaho Indians of Arizona use a form of herbal sauna for the treatment of a variety of diseases including chronic viral infections. Some improvement in the well-being of patients with these chronic viral infections is invariably gained. The various methods of inducing a fever may vary from drugs, vaccines (e.g. BCG vaccine for tuberculosis), exercise, hot packs, steam, hot air, saunas, showers and baths.

The most efficient way of inducing fever is by using either a sauna or a Schlenz bath. In patients with the chronic fatigue syndrome, the application of heat therapies must be approached with caution. The use of drugs and vaccines is definitely forbidden. Expectations from an exercise programme are usually beyond the ability of the sufferer to fulfil them.

The sauna is a steam bath, developed in the Scandinavian countries, that induces a fever resulting in profuse sweating. It is the profuse sweating which is probably of greatest benefit to the CFS sufferer because the sweating process eliminates wastes and toxins from the body. The skin, being the largest organ in the body and having a very large surface area, can act as an efficient eliminating organ. It may even reduce the burden on the kidneys and intestines. It also results in loss of water and electrolytes and these must be replaced in the diet. On the day of the sauna, a patient should consume between three and four litres of water to aid the flushing-out process. Owing to our modern lifestyle, the wearing of clothes and the distinct lack of physical exercise especially in the patient with CFS, the skin's role as a cleansing organ is minimal.

The Schlenz bath is not a recommended detoxification method because it is basically a heating therapy without the production of sweat. Schlenz baths involve the total immersion of the body in a bath of hot water. It is useful though at times of acute viral infections. The Schlenz bath should be hot enough for the patient to bear comfortably without risk of being scalded. The bath should be started at a warm temperature and then hot water added every five to ten minutes to slowly increase the temperature from an initial 95 degrees fahrenheit to 103 degrees fahrenheit. The temperature of both the patient and the water should be monitored and the pulse rate of the patient should not be allowed to rise above 140 beats per minute. If there is any discomfort the patient should be removed from the bath immediately. If possible, bathtime should be approximately one to one and a half hours and it may be performed once or twice a day.

This form of heat therapy can be performed simply and cheaply at home and is indicated as mentioned before only in the CFS patient with an acute viral illness and not in a patient suffering from the chronic fatigue syndrome.

Approximately one third of patients with the chronic fatigue syndrome cannot tolerate any form of heat therapy, including saunas, at all. The reason for this unknown but it is postulated that the heat therapy may itself may stimulate the production of lymphokines (chemicals secreted by the immune system that can cause fatigue) or the heating therapy may actually mobilise stored toxic (xenobiotic chemicals) which pass into the blood stream and affect the nervous system. It is proven scientifically that exercise can mobilise chemicals in this way. If saunas and heat therapy result in an aggravation of the condition, they should be ceased immediately.

It is advisable to use heat therapies at times when the patient can rest immediately afterwards. Heat therapy should be performed on an empty stomach and fresh filtered water or mineral water should be consumed before treatment. The water should be at room temperature and not cold.

Benefits of heat therapies and saunas

1. Stimulate sweating
2. Stimulate waste and toxin removal
3. Increase metabolic processes
4. Increase nervous excitation
5. Relax muscle tension
6. Reduce the motility and secretions of the stomach and intestines
7. Lower the blood pressure
8. May stimulate some hormonal functions
9. Inhibit the growth of viruses
10. Relieve joint pains

Note — as with anything in life, approach the use of saunas and heat therapy with caution and moderation; seek medical advice if you suffer from lung or heart disease.

Exercise

The cardinal symptom in the patient with the chronic fatigue syndrome is muscular tiredness and fatigue after only very slight exertion. Although exercise is the last thing a patient with CFS wants to do, it is an extremely important part of their quest for better health. The motivation to get well, combined with self discipline and some external source of motivation, is essential. An exercise programme may seem daunting to the CFS patient initially but it can be done and done very effectively. The best exercise to commence with is yoga. Yoga is an extremely gentle and non-stressful form of exercise. Even if some yoga postures are tiring, this unwanted side effect is short lived. Yoga breathing exercises contribute to an increase in energy in over two thirds of the CFS patients who have adopted them.

Yoga breathing may be sufficient to start with in an exercise programme, gradually building up to the full yoga exercises and postures. After this has been achieved, brisk walking, light jogging, cycling, swimming and low impact aerobic type exercises may be adopted. The basic rules for the chronic fatigue syndrome patient and exercise is be careful and be moderate. Don't exercise to the point of fatigue. Exercise is meant to improve well-being. A feeling of mild euphoria immediately after exercise sessions should be aimed for.

Two of the most effective yoga postures for the chronic fatigue syndrome sufferer are described here. The first is a posture which is classical — touching the toes. The yogic description of this exercise is that it revitalises the nervous system, stretches the major muscle groups of the back and legs from the head to the feet and massages the contents of the abdomen to reduce constipation, flatulence and acidity. The exercise is simply described as follows:

- Standing as straight and erect as possible, with feet slightly apart, take a deep breath and raise arms high above the head. Bend slowly at the waist bringing the arms down to touch the knees breathing out as you do so. Attempt to stretch down as far as possible with the hands reaching the ankles or feet. Continue breathing out while doing so. Perform the exercise very slowly. Hold the posture for a few seconds and then slowly return to the upright position while inhaling slowly. Repeat this exercise as many times as possible to a total of ten maximum. The slower and more deliberate this exercise is performed, the better are the results. The breathing is extremely important and must be performed slowly and gently.

The second most effective yoga exercise for the chronic fatigue syndrome is the gas-relieving posture, as it is called. This posture again helps in relieving flatulence and stimulates the proper and complete evacuation of the bowels. The exercise is described as follows:

- Lie on the floor on your back with hands straight down beside the hips. Slowly breathing out, bend the legs at the hips raising them to a right angle with the body. Then bend the knees until they come close to or touch the chest and wrap your hands around the legs pulling them in tight against the stomach. Hold the posture for a few seconds and then slowly return to the starting position breathing in very slowly and deliberately as you go.

There are many other postures and yoga exercises that will help individual symptoms but these are best learnt from a trained yoga expert.

Yoga — like meditation, exercise and diet — requires self discipline and deliberation. But it helps even more if there is a genuine desire to get better.

Enjoyable exercise is the key to stress reduction

Once the symptoms of the fatigue syndrome have improved, more vigorous exercise can be commenced cautiously.

Exercise seems to be a particularly desirable method of treatment for stress as it requires very little equipment, is inexpensive and can be done at home. Exercise definitely has no undesirable side effects if performed sensibly and in moderation. Exercise reduces physical stress as well as emotional and mental stresses. It lowers the pulse rate and blood pressure, it improves strength and endurance and it improves the overall fitness of the heart and lungs. Exercise also increases the high density lipoproteins, which are the fats in the blood which help to prevent heart attacks. These substances are also known as HDL-cholesterol, and this is the good form of cholesterol.

A wide range of psychological and emotional benefits result from exercise. These include a reduction in fatigue, greater stamina and vigour, a reduction in depression and anxiety, relaxation of muscular tension and interestingly, a decrease in anger scores. This last benefit is an important reminder to a society of sedentary individuals in which anger manifests itself in violence — perceived to be a growing problem. Furthermore, it has been scientifically shown that there is an increase in clarity of thought and improved concentration as a result of healthy exercise. Aerobic exercise also improves perceptual functioning such as problem-solving ability, short-term memory and 'psychological' speed and reaction time performance.

Proven psychological benefits of exercise

Reduces depression
Decreases anxiety
Improves concentration and clarity of thought
Increases vigour
Decreases fatigue
Relaxes muscular tension
Decreases anger
Positive changes in eating habits, smoking and sexual functioning

The important thing to remember is that exercise must be regular and enjoyable in order to experience its benefits. Unless the exercise is enjoyable, pleasant and regular it may add to your stress. Exercising vigorously and at high intensity is probably more taxing and stressful to most people than longer duration and low intensity exercise, such as walking and yoga. If the high intensity exercise is stressful it is quite likely that there will be little or no improvements in mood, anxiety and depression despite positive gains with regard to weight loss and improved cardiovascular fitness.

We generally see improvement in moods and emotions in people who exercise moderately 20 minutes twice a week for twelve weeks, providing the exercise is enjoyable. No improvements occur if, for example, one jogs in cold wet weather or swims in an excessively hot water swimming pool. Thus exercising in extreme weather conditions, for example hot, cold, wet or humid conditions and so on, may neutralize the effects of exercising and result only in minor mood changes or no improvement at all. Therefore, although jogging and walking are conducive to psychological well-being, cycling at noon on a hot summer's day may result in some cardiovascular benefits but reduce the psychological benefits.

Another very important aspect of exercise is that it should be non-competitive. Competitive sports are important socially and psychologically for other reasons. However, it has been found that competition and competitive activities increase stress. There are always losers and always winners in competitive sports. The winners may feel less stressed, but those who don't win are at greater risk of suffering stress. An effective exercise prescription for stress reduction excludes competition and sports such as football, tennis, basketball and other team sports. Golf, despite player's enthusiasm for it's outdoor and seemingly non-competitive nature, has stressful components to it.

An additional and important requirement in exercise activity is that it is practised regularly and in familiar surroundings. This can be achieved with yoga, simple gymnastics, walking, swimming and jogging. These forms allow you to immediately switch off, tune-out or withdraw from the outside world into your own mental world of imagery. In a way, this is a form of meditation. These activities allow your mind the freedom to wander and reduce attention to the real world. This freedom of the mind seems to be helpful in enhancing the mood and freeing up the emotions. Exercise which is repetitive and rhythmical, such as cycling, jogging, walking, swimming and yoga, seem to be more conducive to producing psychological benefit. Experienced meditators know that repetitive and rhythmical movements, mantras, sounds and breathing are the easy pathways to the meditative state.

Exercise frequency is very important. Exercise should be regular and fit in to your weekly schedule. It should start at a low level and be gentle. Exercising vigorously to begin with is not pleasant and will not give the expected benefits. Taxing, difficult exercises will be neither enjoyable nor stress reducing. Regular training is essential before mood benefits are felt and sedentary people who exercise vigorously without training and building up to a satisfactory exercise level do not achieve psychological benefits.

So, to start with, a ten minute walk in the morning and a ten minute walk in the evening is better than a vigorous twenty minute jog.

You must exercise daily or every second day to reinforce the levels of psychological and physical well-being which you have achieved. It has been shown scientifically that the improved feeling of well-being, relaxation and reduced depression lasts from two to six hours after the exercise.

Inactivity, physical fitness and over-training

Clinically, the vast majority of people who develop the chronic fatigue syndrome have been physically unfit and malnourished at the time of the initial assault by the infection, chemical or drug. Over 80% of patients questioned did not exercise regularly. Less than 30 minutes of low impact type aerobic exercise four times a week puts one in the unfit risk category for not only the chronic fatigue syndrome but other diseases, including cardiovascular disorders, as well. In fact, from the historical evidence available, over 85% of patients in a study of more than 200 people with CFS fell into the 'unfit' category. (Brighthope I.E., 1989.)

A small percentage of CFS sufferers, less than 5%, actually

belonged to an over-trained group. These people were either professional athletes or over-trained for such events as marathons, triathlons and other endurance activities. One of the most difficult aspects in the management of this small group of obsessive individuals is reducing their levels of physical over-activity after they have partially recovered. In the early stages of recovery, when energy levels start to return, athletes in this group start to over-train again and burn themselves out. The message is everything in moderation.

Sunlight, depression and energy levels

Sunlight has been shown to have an effect on the 'master gland' in the middle of the brain called the pineal gland. This gland secretes a hormone called melatonin that influences the hypothalamus and pituitary gland and their hormone secretions from the brain. As a consequence of the changes of the amount of sunlight exposure between different seasons, a condition termed seasonal affective disorder has been coined (SAD). This disorder is associated with winter depression and summer hypomania (over-activity without mania). Patients suffering from SAD are depressed, have low physical and mental energy, over-sleep and feel better on holiday when there is more outdoor activity and presumably more sunlight. Scientific studies have shown that patients with depression and SAD respond to the anti-depressant effects of full-spectrum natural light. The anti-depressant effect is probably caused by the change the circadian (daily) rhythms of melatonin and other hormone synthesis mentioned earlier in the discussion on the timing of meals. Melatonin actually inhibits the secretion of two of the body's stress hormones — ACTH and cortisol. High levels of cortisol are often found in the blood of depressed patients.

It is recommended that exposure to full spectrum light be increased for patients with the CFS to assist with the element of depression. Improved energy levels are achieved in some patients. The exposure must be daily and for those confined indoors the use of proper full-spectrum fluorescent light is advocated. Developing the habit of looking at the light for a few minutes every hour should be encouraged.

Chelation therapy

The word chelate is derived from the Greek word chele which refers to the claw of the crab. The word itself implies a firm pincher like action or binding effect. In biological terms therefore, chelation is the binding of a metal to an organic or inorganic molecule. In chelation therapy we talk about the binding of a chelating substance to heavy metals for example lead, zinc, mercury, cadmium etc. Chelation therapy involves the administration of a chelating substance, called EDTA or Ethylenediaminetetraacetiacid, usually by an intravenous infusion. It is not routinely used in orthodox medicine except for patients with heavy metal poisonings. In the chronic fatigue syndrome it can be demonstrated by full hair analysis that as many as 30% of patients have high levels of heavy metals in their system.

The hair analysis is the most accurate method of measuring these heavy metals and an assessment of the total toxic load of heavy metals can be obtained from this test. If the levels are high, and there has been no response to any other form of therapy, chelation should be seriously considered in the recalcitrant patient. In the right hands, the use of intravenous EDTA, 2 to 3 grams in 500mls of intravenous fluid daily, is extremely safe. Providing the patient has good kidney function, and kidney function is monitored closely, the removal of heavy metals by this method can be extremely rewarding. Vitamins C, B-complex and minerals are given simultaneously. Between three and twenty chelation treatments administered on a daily basis are generally recommended. Some patients may feel an improvement after only three or four chelations. In this group of patients it is recommended that a total of between six and ten treatments are given. It is pointless giving chelation therapy if the source of heavy metal toxification persists. Nothing can be done about the leaching out of lead from the bones into the bloodstream during chelation therapy. However, something can be done about other sources of lead especially if patients live near busy highways where the air is polluted from motor car exhausts. That is, moving to a cleaner environment to reduce the body's burden of lead.

Similarly, the patient with high levels of mercury will only benefit temporarily from chelation therapy if nothing is done about their mercury-silver amalgam dental fillings. Careful removal of dental amalgam fillings by a properly trained dentist using special dams and replacement with modern resins is recommended if mercury levels are high or mercury sensitivity can be demonstrated. Other less significant heavy metals in respect to the chronic fatigue syndrome are cadmium, arsenic and aluminium. However, the presence of these toxic metals even in small amounts can add significant value to the total toxic heavy metal load.

Orthodox immunotherapy

The chronic fatigue syndrome has remained an enigma for orthodox medicine. The exact cause or causes and its pathology have not as yet been accurately defined. Equally, effective treatment by orthodox methods has been a virtual failure. As a consequence, patients have been referred from one medical practitioner to another and to some of the best specialists in the country to no avail. In fact, many have ended up on a psychiatrist's couch with various diagnoses ranging from chronic anxiety, depression, worker's compensation neurosis, various phobias and so on.

This has resulted in frustrated patients — not only with their medical carers, but of the entire health care delivery system. Naturopaths, chiropractors, psychologists and some 'complementary alternative' doctors have, to a large degree, filled this therapeutic gap. By giving appropriate advice regarding changes to lifestyle and, more importantly, advising on the use of nutrient-dense diets, vitamin, mineral and other nutritional supplements and the avoidance of food and chemical sensitivities, the opportunity for greater self-control and management has been provided for many an unfortunate CFS victim. Orthodox medical and psychiatric management are important in the overall care of patients with CFS, but lifestyle changes and natural medicines are the mainstay of treatment.

There are **some** promising approaches on the medical horizon for the treatment of CFS. One of these is the use of intravenous gamma-globulin. A number of clinical trials have been performed supporting the use of gamma-globulin. This is an antibody protein fraction extracted from the plasma or fluid component of human blood. Both physical and psychological benefits from this treatment have been shown and some patients treated with gamma-globulin have shown improvement in their immune system.

High doses of intravenous gamma-globulin are proven to be of benefit and may be even curative in some cases of idiopathic thrombocytopaenia, myasthenia gravis, pemphigus, haemolytic anaemia and other auto-immune diseases. These are all conditions in which the immune system's control mechanisms are disturbed in some way and the immune system produces antibodies to the person's own tissues (i.e. self-antibodies) — biological treason. The use of gamma-globulin may act as a regulator of the immune system and it probably affects the function of suppressor cells.

Another substance that is being used in CFS is transfer factor by intramuscular injection. Transfer factor is protein made from the white cells of healthy people. It has been shown to transfer cell-mediated immunity to patients who have a cell-mediated immune deficiency. The use of transfer factor therefore makes the patient's white blood cells function more effectively reducing infections, infestations, allergies and perhaps even cancer. More work is yet to be done on the importance of transfer factor in CFS.

Another drug that has been tried in CFS is the anti-viral drug, Acyclovir. Anti-viral drugs have not been shown to have any significant benefit in chronic fatigue syndrome. In fact, many drugs which have been trialled in chronic fatigue syndrome have been found to be worthless. Anti-depressants, for example, have actually been shown to exacerbate rather than relieve the symptoms of depression that are associated with the syndrome. This in itself should suggest to the astute clinician that synthetic or xenobiotic chemicals may actually produce hypersensitivity reactions in this group of patients.

In fact any patient — whether they have chronic fatigue syndrome or not — who suffers from mild, moderate or severe side-effects from using synthetic medication should be examined for food and chemical sensitivities. Their vitamin, mineral, trace element and anti-oxidant status should be carefully assessed. There is good scientific evidence now to suggest that this group of sensitive patients are at greater risk of developing severe disease such as heart disease, hypertension, diabetes, arthritis, stroke, asthma, emphysema and perhaps even some forms of cancer. Dietary supplements invariably help them.

Included in this section on orthodox immunotherapy is a brief mention of the use of intravenous vitamin C therapy. This is discussed at greater length elsewhere in this book. However, it is mentioned here because there is a growing number of medical practitioners and specialists in this country who are using megadose intravenous vitamin C therapy very effectively in the management of CFS. It must be emphasised here that the earlier the treatment with intravenous vitamin C the better the result. Even with long-standing CFS cases the results are very good, but it may take longer for them to be achieved.

References

Chapter 1

E.D. Acheson, 'The clinical syndrome variously called benign myalgic encephalomyelitis, Iceland disease and epidemic neuromyasthenia' (1970) *Am J Med* 1:7-11.

Anonymous. 'A new clinical entity?' (1956) *Lancet* editorial 1:789-90.

Anonymous. 'Epidemic myalgic encephalomyelitis' (1978) *Br Med J* 1:1436-7.

P.O. Behan, W.M.H. Behan, E.J. Bell, 'The post-viral fatigue syndrome: an analysis of the findings in 50 cases' (1985) *J Infection* 10:211-22.

E. Byrne, 'Chronic myalgia, a personal approach' (1986) *Aust NZ J Med* 16:745-48.

E. Byrne, 'Idiopathic chronic fatigue and myalgia syndrome some thoughts on nomenclature and aetiology' (1988) *Med J Aust* 148:80-2.

A. Gilliam, 'Epidemiological study of an epidemic diagnosed as poliomyelitis occurring among the personnel of the Los Angeles County Hospital during the summer of 1934' (1938) *Public Health Bull* 240.

G. Holmes, J. Kaplan, N. Gantz et al, 'Chronic fatigue syndrome: a working case definition' (1988) *Ann Intern Med* 108:387-9.

A. Lloyd, D. Wakefield, C. Boughton, J. Dwyer, 'What is myalgic encephalomyelitis?' (1988) *Lancet* 1:1286-7.

C.P. McEvedy, A.W. Beard, 'Concept of benign myalgic encephalomyelitis' (1970) *Br Med J* 1:11-15.

C.P. McEvedy, A.W. Beard, 'Royal Free epidemic of 1955: a reconsideration' (1970) *Br Med J* 1:7-11.

Medical Staff Royal Free Hospital, 'An outbreak of encephalomyelitis in the Royal Free Hospital Group, London in 1955' (1957) *Br Med J* 2:895-904.

R.A. Pellew, J.A.R. Miles, 'Further investigations on a disease resembling poliomyelitis seen in Adelaide' (1955) *Med J Aust* 2:480-5.

Chapter 2

H. Beckman, 'Phenylalanine in affective disorders' (1983) *Adv Biol Psychiat* 10:137-47.

A. Bennett, R. Doll and R. Howell, 'Sugar consumption and cigarette smoking' (1970) *Lancet* 1:1011-4.

P. Bermond, 'Therapy of side effects of oral contraceptive agents with vitamin B6' (1982) *Acta Vitaminol-Enzymol* 4:45-54.

J. Blair, C. Morar, C. Hamon et al, 'Tetrahydrobiopterin metabolism in depression' (1984) *Lancet* 1:163.

S. Bolton, G. Null, 'Caffeine, psychological effects, use and abuse' (1981) *J Orthomol Psychiatry* 10:202-11.

K.W. Bridges, D.P. Goldberg, 'Psychiatric illness in patients with neurological disorders: patients' views on discussion of emotional problems with neurologists' (1984) *Br Med J* 289:656-58.

M. Brook, J. Grimshaw, 'Vitamin C concentration of plasma and leukocytes as related to smoking habit, age and sex of humans' (1968) *Am J Clin Nutr* 21:1254-8.

R. Brown, 'Tryptophan metabolism in humans', in O. Hayaishi, Y. Ishimura, R. Kido (eds), *Biochemical and Medical Aspects of Tryptophan Metabolism* (Elsevier/-North Holland Press, Amsterdam, 1980, pp.227-36).

R. Buckley, 'Hypoglycemic kindling of limbic system disorder' (1978) *J Orthomol Psychiatry* 7:118-22.

R. Buist, 'The therapeutic predictability of tryptophan and tyrosine in the treatment of depression' (1983) *Int J Clin Nutr Rev* 3:1-3.

M. Carney, B. Sheffield, 'Associations of subnormal folate and B12 values and effects of replacement therapy' (1970) *J Nerv Ment Dis* 150:404-12.

M. Carney, D. Williams, B. Sheffield, 'Thiamin and pyridoxine lack in newly-admitted psychiatric patients' (1979) *Br J Psychiatry* 135:249-54.

G. Chouinard et al, 'Tryptophan in the treatment of depression and mania' (1983) *Adv Biol Psychiat* 10:47-66.

H. Curtius, A. Niederwieser, R. Levine et al, 'Successful treatment of depression with tetrahydrobiopterin' (1983) *Lancet* 1:657-8.

H. Curtius, H. Muldner, A. Niederwieser, 'Tetrahydrobiopterin. Efficacy in endogenous depression and Parkinson's disease' (1982) *J Neural Trans* 55:301-8.

D. Evans, G. Edelsohn, R. Golden, 'Organic psychosis without anemia or spinal cord symptoms in patients with vitamin B12 deficiency' (1983) *Am J Psychiatry* 140:218-21.

C. Gibson, 'Control of monoamine synthesis by amino acid precursors' (1983) *Adv Biol Psychiat* 10:4-18.

F. Goggans, 'A case of mania secondary to vitamin B12 deficiency' (1984) *Am J Psychiatry* 141:300-1.

J. Greden, P. Fontaine, M. Lubetsky, K. Chamberlian, 'Anxiety and depression associated with caffeinism among psychiatric patients' (1979) 131:1089-94.

J. Growden, 'Neurotransmitter precursors in the diets: their use in the treatment of brain diseases' in R. Wurtman, J. Wurtman (eds), *Nutrition and the Brain* (Raven Press, New York, NY, 1979, vol. 3, pp.117-82).

I. Hickie, A. Lloyd, D. Wakefield, G. Parker, 'The psychiatric status of patients with chronic fatigue syndrome' (1990) *Br J Psychiatry* 156:534-40.

B. Hunter, 'Some food additives as neuroexcitors and neurotoxins' (1984) *Clinical Ecology* 2:83-9.

D. Johnson, K. Dorr, W. Swenson, J. Service, 'Reactive hypoglycemia' (1980) *JAMA* 243:1151-5.

D. King, 'Can allergic exposure provoke psychological symptoms? A double-blind test' (1981) *Biol Psychiatry* 16:3-19.

R. Kinsman and J. Hood, 'Some behavioral effects of ascorbic acid deficiency ' (1971) *Am J Clin Nutr* 24:455-64.

M. Krause, L. Mahan, *Food, Nutrition and Diet Therapy* (W.B. Saunders Co., Philadelphia, Pa, 1984).

M.J.P. Kruesi, J. Dale, S. Straus, 'Psychiatric diagnoses in patients who have chronic fatigue syndrome' (1989) *J Clin Psychiatry* 50:53-6.

H. Landmann, R. Sutherland, 'Incidence and significance of pypoglycemia in unselected admissions to a psychosomatic service' (1950) *Am J Dig Dis* 17:105-8.

R.B. Layzer, L.P. Rowland, I.M. Ranney, 'Muscle phosphofructokinase deficiency' (1967) *Arch Neurol* 17:512-23.

R. Leeming, J. Harpey, S. Brown, J. Blair, 'Tetrahydrofolate and hydroxycobolamin in the management of Dihydropteridine reductase deficiency' (1982) *J Ment Def Res* 26:21-5.

K. Lindstrom, H. Riihimaki, K. Hanninen, 'Occupational solvent exposure and neuropsychiatric disorders' (1984) *Scan J Work Environ Health* 10:321-3.

M. Lipton, R. Maiman, C. Nemeroff, 'Vitamins, megavitamin therapy and the nervous system' in R. Wurtman, J. Wurtman (eds), *Nutrition and the Brain* (Raven Press, New York, NY, 1979, vol. 3, pp.183-264).

A. Niems, R. von Borstel, 'Caffeine: metabolism and biochemical mechanisms of action' in R. Wurtman, J. Wurtman (eds), *Nutrition and the Brain* (Raven Press, New York, NY, 1983, vol. 6, pp.2-30).

B. Nobbs, 'Pyridoxal phosphate status in clinical depression' (1974) *Lancet* 1:405.

J. Olsen, S. Sabroe, 'A case-reference study of neuropsychiatric disorders among workers exposed to solvents in the Danish wood and furniture industry' (1980) *Scand J Soc Med suppl* 16:34-43.

W. Pardridge, 'Regulation of amino acid availability to the brain' in R. Wurtman, J. Wurtman (eds), *Nutrition and the Brain*, Raven Press, New York, NY, vol. 1, pp.142-204).

O. Pelletier, 'Smoking and vitamin C levels in humans' (1968) *Am J Clin Nutr* 21:1259-67.

E. Reynolds, J. Preece, J. Bailey, A. Coppen, 'B12 deficiency in depressive illness' (1970) *Br J Psychiat* 117:287-92.

H. Salzer, 'Reactive hypoglycemia as a cause of neuropsychiatric illness' (1966) *J Nat Med Assoc* 58:12 7.

T. Sourkes, 'Nutrients and the cofactors required for monoamine synthesis in nervous tissue' in R. Wurtman, J. Wurtman (eds) *Nutrition and the Brain* (Raven Press, New York, NY, 1979, vol.3, pp.265-99).

J.W. Stewart, W. Harrison, F. Quitkin, H. Baker, 'Low level B6 levels in depressed outpatients' (1984) *Biolog Psychiat* 19:613-6.

G.S. Taerk, B.B. Toner, I.E. Salit et al, 'Depression in patients with neuromyasthenia (benign myalgic encephalomyelitis)' (1987), *Int J Psychiatry* 17:49-56.

V. Wynn, P. Adams, J. Folkard, M. Seed, 'Tryptophan, depression and steriodal contraception' (1975) *J. Steroid Biochem* 6:965-70.

D. Zucker, R. Livingstone, R. Nakra, P. Clayton, 'B12 deficiency and psychiatric disorders: a case report and literature review' (1981) *Biol psychiatry* 16:197-205.

Chapter 3

J.E. Abraham, C.W. Svare, C.W. Frank, 'The effect of dental amalgam restoration on blood mercury levels' (1984) *J Dent Res* 63:71-3.

Ahlrot-Westerlund (1985) *Nutr Res, suppl* 403. Second Nordic symp on trace elements in human health and disease, Odense, Denmark, Aug 1987.

D.L. Arnold, P.J. Bore, G.K. Radda et al, 'Excessive intra-

REFERENCES

cellular acidosis of skeletal muscle on exercise in a patient with a post-viral exhaustion/-fatigue syndrome.' A P nuclear magnetic resonance study (1984) *Lancet* 1:1367-9.

P. Bloch, I.M. Shapiro, Summary of the international conference on mercury hazards in dental practice (1982) *J Amer Dent Assoc* 104:489-90.

E. Byrne, I. Trounce, 'Oxygen electrode studies with human skeletal muscle mitochondria in vitro. A reappraisal' (1985) *J Neurol Sci* 69:319-33.

L.W. Chang, 'Neurotoxic effects of mercury — a review' (1977) *Environ Res* 14:329-73.

T.W. Clarkson, 'Biochemical aspects of mercury poisoning' (1968) *J Occup Med* 10:351-55.

T.W. Clarkson, L. Friberg, J. Hursh, M. Mylander in *Biological monitoring of toxic metals* (Plenum Press, NY, Feb 1988).

W. Craelius, 'Comparative epidemiology of multiple sclerosis and dental caries' (1978) *J Epidemiol Comm Hlth* 32:155 65.

G. Czapsk, J. Aronovitch, M. Chevion, 'On the mechanisms of cytotoxicity induced by superoxide' in *Oxygen radicals in chemistry and biology* (Walter de Gruyter and Co., Berlin, New York, printed in Germany, 1984).

E. Dejarassi, N. Berova, 'The possibilities of allergic reactions from silver amalgam restorations' (1969) *Int Den J* 19:481-88.

David D.D.S. Eggleston, 'Effect of dental amalgam and nickel alloys on T-lymphocytes' (May 1984) Preliminary report, *J Prosthetic Dentistry*, vol.51,no.5:617-23.

EPA Mercury health effects update health issue assessment (1984), Final report EPA-600¾4-8-84-019F, United States Environmental Protection Agency, Office of Health and Environment Assessment, Wash DD 20460.

D.D. Gay, R.D. Cox, J.W. Reinhardt, 'Chewing releases mercury from fillings' (1979) *Lancet* 1:984-5.

L.J. Goldwater, 'The toxicology of inorganic mercury' (1957) *Annals NY Acad Sci* 65:498-503.

H. Gordon, 'Pregnancy in female dentists — a mercury hazard' (Sept 1981) in proceedings of Internat Conf on mercury hazards in dental practice, Glasgow, Scotland, 2-4.

H. Huggins, 'Mercury — a factor in mental disease?" (1982) *J of Orthomolec Psych* 11(1):3-16.

H.A. Huggins, 'It's all in your head' (1985) Toxic Element Research Foundation, Colorado Springs, CO.

J.B. Hursh, T.W. Clarkson, M.G. Cherian, J.J. Vostall, Millie A. Vander, 'Clearance of mercury (Hg-197, Hg-203) vapour inhaled by human subjects' (1976) *Arch Environ Hlth* 31:302-9.

G.A. Jamal, S. Hansen, 'Electrophysiological studies in patients with post-viral fatigue syndrome' (1985) *J Neurol Neurosurg Psychiatry* 48:691-4.

B. Koos, L. Longo, 'Mercury toxicity in the pregnant woman, fetus and newborn infant' (1976) *Am J Obstet Gynec*.

Kuntz, (1982) *Am J Obst and Gynecol* 143:440-43.

E.S. Lain, G.S. Caughron, 'Electrogalvanic phenomena of the oral cavity caused by dissimilar metalic restorations' (1936) *JADA* 23:1641-45.

O. Lamm, H. Pratt, 'Subclinical effects of exposure to inorganic mercury revealed by somatosensory-evoked potentials' (1985) *Eur Neurol* 24:237-43.

G. Macdonald, 'Occupational hazards in dentistry' (1984) *J Calif Dent Assoc* 12:17-19.

M. Nakamura, H. Kawahara, 'Cellular response to the dispersion amalgams' (1979) *J Dent Res* 58:1780-90.

Magnus Nylander, Lars Friberg, Berger Lind, 'Mercury concentrations in human brain and kidneys in relation to exposure from dental amalgam fillings' (1987) *Swed Dent J* 11:179-87.

M. Nylander, 'Mercury in pituitary glands of dentists' (1986) *Lancet* 22 Feb 442.

J. Pleva, 'Mercury poisoning from dental amalgams' (1983) *J Orthomolec Psych* 12:184-93.

H.Raue, 'Resistance to therapy; think of tooth fillings.' (1980) *Med Prac* 32:2303-9.

S. Ribarov, L. Benov, I. Benchev, 'HgC12 increases the methemoglobin peroxidant activity. Possible mechanism of Hg2¢ induced lipid peroxidation in erythrocytes' (1984) *Chem Biol Interac* 50:111-19.

A. Rothstein, 'Cell membrane as site of action of heavy metals' (1959) *Fed Proc* 18:1026-35.

R.S. Schottenfeld, M.R. Cullen, 'Organic affective illness associated with lead intoxication' (1984) *Am J Psychiat* 141:1423-6.

Sharma and Obersteiner, 'Metals and neurotoxic effects; cytotoxicity of selected compounds on chick ganglia cultures' (1981) *J of Comparative Pathology* 91:235-44.

C.W. Svare, L. Peterson et al, 'The effect of dental amalgams on mercury levels in expired air' (1981) *J Dental Research* vol.60, no.9:1668-71.

C.W. Svare, L. Peterson, 'The effect removing dental

amalgam on mercury blood levels' (1984) *J Dent Res*, IADR Abst 896.

I.M. Trachtenberg, 'Chronic effects of mercury on organisms' (1974) US Department of Health, National Institute of Health, Bethesda, Maryland.

M.J. Vimy, F.L. Lorscheider, 'Serial measurements of intra oral air mercury: estimation of daily dose from dental amalgam' (Aug 1985) *J Dental Research* vol.64, no.8:1072075.

R.A. Ware, L.W. Chang, P.M. Burkholder, 'An ultrasonic study on the blood-brain barrier dysfunction following mercury intoxification' (1972) *Acta Neuropath* (Berlin) 21:179 84.

S. Ziff, *Silver dental fillings — the toxic time bomb* (Aurora Press, New York, NY, 1984, 1986).

Chapter 4

L.C. Archard, N.E. Bowles, D. Doyle, E. Bell, P. Behan, 'Postviral fatigue syndrome: persistence of enterovirus RNA in muscle and elevated creatine kinase' (1988) *J Royal Soc Med* 81:326-29.

I.E. Brighthope, *The Aids Fighters* (Biocentres, 1987).

I.E. Brighthope, 'The role of nutritional medicine in general practice', *Aust Family Phys*

D. Buchwald, D.L. Goldenberg, J.L. Sullivan, A.L. Komaroff, 'The "chronic, active Epstein-Barr virus infection" syndrome and primary fibromyalgia' (1987), *Arthritis Rheum* 30: 1132-36.

E. Byrne, I. Trounce, 'Chronic fatigue and myalgia syndrome: mitochondrial and glycolytic studies in skeletal muscle' (1987) *J Neurol Neurosurg Psychiatry* 50:743-47.

E. Byrne, I. Trounce, X Dennett, 'Chronic relapsing myalgia (?postviral): clinical, histological and biochemical studies' (1985) *Aust NZ J Med* 15:305-8.

E. Byrne, J.F. Hallpike, P.C. Blumbergs, T.M. Mukherjee, 'Clinical features of mitochondrial myopathy' (1983) *Aust NZ J Med* 13:353-8.

E. Byrne, I. Trounce, 'Chronic fatigue and myalgia syndrome: mitochondrial and glycolytic studies in skeletal muscle' (1985) *J Neurol Neurosurg Psychiatry* 50:743-6.

E. Byrne, 'Historical and current concepts in mitochondrial myopathies' (1983) *Aust NZ J Med* 13:299-305.

M. Caliguiri, C. Murray, D. Muchwald et al, 'Phenotypic and functional deficiency of natural killer cells in patients with chronic fatigue syndrome' (1987), *J Immunol* 139:3306 3313.

W. Hellinger, T. Smith, R. Van Scoy, P. Spitzer, P. Forgacs, R. Edson, 'Chronic fatigue syndrome and the diagnostic utility of Epstein-Barr virus early antigen' (1988) *J Amer Med Assoc* 260:971-3.

A. Linde, L. Hammarstrom, C. Smith, 'IgG subclass deficiency and chronic fatigue syndrome' (1988) *Lancet* 1:885-6.

A. Lloyd, D. Wakefield, C. Boughton, J. Dwyer, 'Immunological abnormalities in the chronic fatigue syndrome' (1989) *Med J Aust* 151:122-4.

A. Lloyd, J. Hales, S. Gandevia, 'Muscle strength, endurance and recovery in the post infection fatigue syndrome' (1988) *J Neurol Neurosurg Psychiatry* 51:1316-22.

A. Lloyd, D. Wakefield, L. Smith et al, 'Red blood cell morphology in chronic fatigue syndrome' (1989) *Lancet* II:217.

E.M. McDonald, A.H. Mann, H.C. Thomas, 'Interferons as mediators of psychiatric morbidity. An investigation in a trial of recombinant alpha interferon in hepatitis-B carriers' (1987) *Lancet* II:1175-8.

C. McEvedy, A. Beard, 'Concept of benign myalgic encephalomyelitis' (1970) *Br Med J* 1:11-15.

T. Mukherjee, K. Smith, K. Maros, 'Abnormal red blood cell morphology in myalgic encephalomyelitis' (1987) *Lancet* II:328-9.

J. C. Murdoch, 'Cell-mediated immunity in patients with myalgic encephalomyelitis syndrome' (1988) *New Zealand Med J* 101:511-2.

J. Murdoch, 'Myalgic encephalomyelitis (ME) syndrome — an analysis of the findings in 200 cases' (1976) *NZ Family Physician* 14:51-4.

R. Pellew, 'A clinical description of a disease resembling poliomyelitis seen in Adelaide 1949-51.' (1951) *Med J Aust* 1:944.

A. Ramsay, 'Epidemic neuromyasthenia 1955-1978' (1978) *Postgrad Med J* 54:718-21.

R. Read, G. Spickett, J. Harvey, A. Edwards, H. Larson, 'IgG1 sublcass deficiency in patients with chronic fatigue syndrome' (1988) *Lancet* 1:241.

M. Stokes, R.G. Cooper, R.H.T. Edwards, 'Normal muscle strength and fatiguability in patients with effort syndromes' (1988) *Br Med J* 297:1014-7.

S.E. Straus, J.K. Dale, M. Tobi et al, 'Acyclovir treatment of the chronic fatigue syndrome: lack of efficacy in a placebo controlled trial' (1988) *N Engl J Med* 319:1692-8.

S. Straus, G. Tosato, G. Armstrong et al, 'Persisting illness and fatigue in adults with evidence of Epstein-Barr virus infection' (1985) *Ann*

Intern Med 102:7-16.

D. Wakefield, A. Lloyd, J. Dwyer, S. Salahuddin, D. Ablashi, 'Human herpesvirus 6 and myalgic encephalomyelitis' (1988) *Lancet* 1:146-50.

D. Wakefield, A. Lloyd, 'Pathophysiology of myalgic encephalomyelitis' (1987) *Lancet* II:918-9.

R.P. Yonge, 'Magnetic resonance muscle studies: implications for psychiatry' (1988) *J Royal Soc Med* 81:322-5.

G. Yousef, E. Bell, G. Mann et al, 'Chronic enterovirus infection in patients with post-viral fatigue syndrome' (1988) *Lancet* 1:146-50.

Chapter 5

J.D. Balentine, *Pathology of Oxygen Toxicity* (1982, Academic Press, New York).

A.A. Barber, 'Mechanisms of lipid peroxide formation in rat tissue homogenates' (1963) *Radiat Res* suppl.3:33-43.

A.A. Barber, F. Bernheim, 'Lipid peroxidation: its measurement, occurence and significance in animal tissues' (1967) *Adv Gerontol Res* 2:355-403.

E. Beutler, 'Glucose 6 phosphate dehydrogenase deficiency and red cell glutathione peroxidase' (1977) *Blood* 49:467-9.

E.J. Calabrese, *Nutrition and Environmental Health* (1980, John Wiley, New York, vol.1).

D. Chiu, B. Lubin, S.B. Shohet, 'Peroxidative reactions in red cell biology' in W.A. Prior (ed), *Free Radicals in Biology* (Academic Press, New York, 1982, vol.5, pp.115-9).

C.K. Chow, 'Influence of dietary vitamin E on susceptibility to ozone exposure' in S.D. Lee, M.G. Mustafa, M.A. Mehlman (eds) *The biomedical effects of ozone and related photochemical oxidants - proceedings of an international symposium* (1982, Princeton Scientific Publishers, Princeton, NJ, pp.75-94).

H.B. Demopoulos et al, 'Oxygen free radicals in central nervous system ischemia and trauma' in A.P. Autor (ed) *Pathology and Oxygen* (1982, Academic Press, New York, pp.127-55.

C.J. Dillard et al, 'Effects of exercise, vitamin E and ozone on pulmonary function and lipid peroxidation' (1978) *J Appl Physiol* 45:927-32.

A.T. Diplock, 'Metabolic and functional defects in selenium deficiency' (1981) *Phil Trans R Soc Lond* B294:105-17.

L. Flohe, 'Glutathione peroxidase brought into focus' in W.A. Pryor (ed) *Free Radicals in Biology* (1982, Academic Press, New York, vol.5, pp.223-54).

H.J. Forman, E.I. Rotman, A.B. Fisher, 'Role of selenium and sulfur-containing amino acids in protection against oxygen toxicity' (1983) *Lab.Invest* 49:148-53.

H.J. Forman, A. Boveris, 'Superoxide radical and hydrogen peroxide in mitochondria' in W.A. Pryor (ed.) *Free Radicals in Biology* (1982, Academic Press, New York, vol.5, pp.65 89).

I. Fridovich, 'Superoxide dismutase in biology and medicine' in A.P. Autor (ed) *Pathology of Oxygen* (Academic Press, New York, 1982, pp.1-20).

I. Fridovich, 'Superoxide radical: an endogenous toxicant' (1983) *Ann Rev Pharmacol Toxicol* 23:239-57.

J. Glavind et al, 'Studies on the role of lipoperoxides in human pathology. 2. The presence of peroxidized lipids in the atherosclerotic aorta' (1952) *Acta Pathol* 30:1-6.

W.J. Goodwin et al, 'Selenium and glutathione peroxidase levels in patients with epidermoid carcinoma of the oral cavity and oropharynx' (1983) *Cancer* 51:110-15).

K. Grankvist, S. Marklund, I.B. Taljedal, 'Superoxide dismutase is a prophylactic against alloxan diabetes' (1981) *Nature* 294:158-60.

A.C. Griffin, H.W. Lane, 'Selenium chemoprevention of cancer in animals and possible human implications' in J.E. Spallholz, J.L. Martin, H.E. Ganther (ed) *Selenium in Biology and Medicine* — proceedings of 2nd international symposium (1981, AVI Publishing, Westport CT, pp.160-170).

J.M.C. Gutteridge, J. Stocks, 'Peroxidation of cell lipids' (1976) *Med Lab Sci* 33:281-5.

J.D. Hackney et al, 'Experimental studies on human health effects of air pollutants: II Ozone Arch.' (1975) *Environ Hlth* 30:379-84.

D.G. Hafeman, W.G. Hoekstra, 'Protection against carbon tetrachloride-induced lipid peroxidation in the rat by dietary vitamin E, selenium and methionine as measure by ethane evolution' *J Nutr* 107:656-65.

B. Halliwell, J.M.C. Gutteridge, *Free radicals in biology and medicine* (Oxford: Clarendon Press, 1984).

D. Harman, 'The ageing process' (1981) *Proc Natl Acad Sci USA* 78:7124-8.

A. Hoffer, 'Oxidation-reduction and the brain' (1983) *J Orthomol Psych* 12:292-301.

L. Johlin et al, 'Glood glutathione peroxidase levels in skin diseases: effects of selenium and vitamin E treatment' (1982) *Acta Dermatol Verereol* 62:211-4.

H. Kappus, H. Sies, 'Toxic drug effects associated with

oxygen metabolism. Redox cycling and lipid peroxidation' (1981) *Experientia* 37:1233-41.

S.A. Levine, J.H. Reinhardt, 'Biochemical pathology initiated by free radicals, oxidant chemicals and therapeutic drugs in the etiology of chemical hypersensitivity disease' (1983) *J Orthomol Psych* 12:166-83.

R.P. Mason, C.F. Chignell, 'Free radicals in pharmacology and toxicology — selected topics' (1983) *Pharmacol* 33:189 211.

D.C.H. McBrien, T.F. Slater (eds), *Free radicals, lipid peroxidation and cancer* (1982, Academic Press, London).

A.M. Michelson, 'Clinical use of superoxide dismutase and possible pharmacological approaches' in A.P. Autor (ed) *Pathology of Oxygen* (Academic Press, New York, 1982, pp.277-302).

H.P. Misra, I. Fridovich, 'The role of superoxide anion in the autooxidation of epinephrine and a simple assay for superoxide dismutase' (1972) *J Biol Chem* 247:3170-5.

R.H. Pain, 'Dressing the SOD' (1983) *Nature* 306:228.

G. Perona et al, 'In vivo and in vitro variations of human erythrocyte glutatione peroxidase activity as result of cells aging, selenium availability and peroxidase activation' (1978) *Br J Haematol* 39:399-408.

D. Pessayre et al, 'Effect of fasting on metabolite-mediated hepatotoxicity in the rat' (1979) *Gastroenterol* 77:264 171.

W.A. Pryor, 'Free radical biology: xenobiotics, cancer and aging' (1982) *Ann NY Acad Sci* 393:1-22.

W.J. Rea, 'Environmentally triggered cardiac disease' (1978) *Ann Allergy* 40:243-51.

J.B. Schenkman et al, 'Active oxygen in liver microsomes: mechanism of epinephrine oxidation' (1979) *Mol Pharmacol* 15:428-38.

M.T. Smith, H. Thor, S. Orrenius, 'The role of lipid peroxidation in the toxicity of foreign compounds to liver cells' (1983) *Biochem Parmacol* 32:763-4.

J.E. Spalholz, 'Selenium: what role in immunity and immune cytotoxicity?' in J.E., Spalholz, J.L. Martin and H.E. Ganther (eds) *Selenium in Biology and Medicine* — proceedings of 2nd international symposium (AVI Publishing, Westport CT, 1981, pp.103-117).

H.F. Stokinger, L.D. Scheel, 'Ozone toxicity: immunochemical and tolerance producing aspects' (1962) *Arch Environ Hlth* 4:327-334.

M. Suthanthiran, S.D. Solomon, P.S. Williams, A.L. Rubin, A. Novogrodsky, K.H. Stenzel, 'Hydroxyl radical scavengers inhibit human natural killer cell activity' (1984) *Nature* 307:276-8.

A.L. Tappel, 'Measurement of and protection from in vivo lipid peroxidation' in W.A. Pryor (ed) *Free Radicals in Biology* (Academic Press, New York, 1980, vol.4,pp.2-47).

A.L. Tappel, 'Measurement of in vivo lipid peroxidation via exhaled pentane and protection by vitamin E' in K. Yagi (ed) *Lipid Peroxides in Biology and Medicine* (Academic Press, New York, 1982, pp.213-22).

A.I. Tauber, N. Borregaard, E. Simons, J. Wright, 'Chronic granulomatous disease: a syndrome of phagocyte oxidase deficiencies' (1983) *Medicine* 62:286-309.

A.J. Vander, *Nutrition, Stress and Toxic Chemicals* (1981, university of Michigan Press, Ann Arbor).

J.F. Wilkins, 'Haemoglobin oxidation in whole blood samples from sheep in relation to clutathione peroxidase activity' (1979) *Austral J Biol Sci* 32:451-6.

H. Witschi, 'Environmental agents altering lung biochemistry' (1977) *Fed Proc* 36:1631-4.

G.K. York et al, 'Stimulation by cigarette smoke of glutathione peroxidase system enzyme activities in rat lung' (1976) *Environ Hlth* 31:286-90.

Chapter 6

D.J. Atherton et al, 'A double-blind controlled crossover trial of an antigen-avoidance diet in atopic eczema' (1978) *Lancet* 1.

R. Buckley, 'Food allergy' (1982) *JAMA* 248-2627.

W.A. Commings, E.W. Williams, 'Transport of large breakdown products of dietary protein through the gut wall' (1978) *Gut* 19:715.

R. Cornell, W.A. Walker, K.J. Isselbacher, 'Small intestinal absorption of horseradish peroxidase' (1981) *Lab Invest* 25:42.

Al de Weck, 'Pathophysiologic mechanisms of allergic and pseudo-allergic reations to foods, food additives and drugs' (1984) *Ann All* 53:583-6.

W.W. Duke, 'Food allergy as a cause of abdominal pain' (1921) *Arch Intern Med* 28-151.

W.W. Duke, 'Meniere's syndrome caused by allergies' (1923) *JAMA* 81-2179.

J. Egger, P.J. Graham, C.M. Carter, D. Gumley, 'Controlled trial of oliogoantigenic treatment in the hyperkinetic syndrome' (1985) *Lancet* 1:540.

J.W. Gerrard, C.G. Ko, P. Vickers, 'The familial incidence of allergic disease' (1976) *Ann All* 36-10.

F.L. Grusky, 'Gastrointestinal absorption of unaltered proteins in normal infants' (1955) *Pediatrics* 16:763.

D.F. Horrobin et al, 'The nutritional regulation of T lymphocyte function' (1979) *Med Hypothesis* 5:969.

S.E. Keller, J.M. Weiss, S.J. Schleifer et al, 'Suppression of immunity by stress: effect of graded series of stressors on lymphocyte stimulation in the rat' (1981) *Science* 213:1397.

A.M. Lake, K.J. Bloch, M.R. Neutra, W.A. Waker, 'Intestinal goblet cell mucous release' (1979) *J Immunol* 122:834.

S.A. Levine, 'Selenium and human chemical hypersensitivities' (1982) *Int J Biosocial* 3:44.

J.J. McGovern, 'Correlation of clinical food allergy symptoms with serial pharmacological and immunological changes in the patient's plasma' (1980) *Ann Allergy* 44-57.

J.D. Minor, S.G. Tolber, O.L. Frick, 'Leukocyte inhibition factor in delayed-onset food sensitivity' (1980) *J Allergy Clin Immunol* 6:314.

J. Monroe, C. Carini, J. Brostoff, Zilkha, 'Food allergy in migraine' (1980) *Lancet* II:1.

B.K. Nandi, N. Subramanian, K. Majumder, L.B. Chatterjee, 'Effect of ascorbic acid on detoxification of histamine under stress conditions' (1974) *Biochem Parmacol* 23:643.

R. Pagnelli, R.J. Levinsky, D.J. Atherton, 'Detection of specific antigen within circulating immune complexes' (1979) *Lancet* 1:1270.

F.L. Pearce, A.D. Befus, J. Bienenstock, 'Effect of quercetin and other flavonoids on antigen-induced histamine secretion from rat intestinal mast cells' (June 1984) *J All Clin Immunol* 822.

R.S. Pekarek, H.H. Sandstead, R.A. Jacob, D.F. Barcome, 'Abnormal cellular immune responses during acquired zinc deficiency' (1979) *Am J Clin Nut* 32:1466.

L. Perelmutter, 'Non-IgE mediated atopic disease' (1984) *Ann All* 52:640.

M.C. Reinhardt, 'Macromolecular absorption of food antigens in health and disease' (1984) *J Allergy* 53:597.

A.H. Rowe, E.J. Young, 'Bronchial asthma due to food allergy alone in 95 patients' (1959) *JAMA* 169:1158.

E. Thonnard-Nenmann, L. Neckers, 'T-lymphocytes in migraine' (1981) *Ann All* 47:325.

R.J. Trevino, 'Immunologic mechanisms in the production of food sensitivities' (1981) *Laryngoscope* 91:1913.

W.A. Walker, 'Uptake and transport of macromolecules by the intestine - possible role in clinical disorders' (1974) *Gastroen* 67:531.

Chapter 7

R. Anderson, *Ascorbic acid and immune function: mechanisms of immuno stimulation — Vitamin C Ascorbic Acid* (Applied Science Publishers, 1981, pp.249-72, by Counsell & Hornig).

R. Anderson, 'Ascorbate mediated stimulation of neutrophil motility and lymphocyte transformation by inhibition of the peroxidase H202 halide system in vitro and in vivo' (1981) *Am J of Clin Nutr* 34:1906-11.

D. Baetgen, 'Results of treatment of epidemic hepatitis in children with high doses of ascorbic acid in the years 1957 to 1959' (1961) *Medinzinische Monatschrift* 15:30-6.

J.C. Bauernfeind, 'The safe use of Vitamin A' (1980) *A report of the International Vitamin A Consultative Groups (IVACC)*, The Nutrition Foundation, Washington.

W.A. Baumgartnea, 'Antioxidants, cancer and the immune response — trace metals in health and disease' (Raven Press, 1979).

H. Baur, H. Staub, 'Hepatitis therapy with infusions of ascorbic acid' (1954) *Schweiz Med Wochenschrift* 84:594 600.

H. Baur, 'Treatment of poliomyelitis with ascorbic acid' (1952) *Helvetia Media Acta* 19:470-74.

W.R. Beisel, 'Single nutrients and immunity' (1982) *Am J of Clin Nutr* 35:417-68 (Suppl).

A. Berger, H.H. Schaumburg, 'More on neuropathy from pyridoxine abuse' (1984) *N Engl J Med* 311:986-7.

E. Cameron, L. Pauling, *Cancer and Vitamin C* (Warner, 1979, pp.96 120, 183-9, 199-203).

R.F. Cathcart, 'The method of determining proper doses of vitamin C for the treatment of disease by titrating to bowel tolerance' (1981) *J Ortho Psych* 10:125-31.

P. Cilento, *You Can't Live Without Vitamin C* (Witcomb and Tombs, 1979, pp.42-44, 71-80, 94-102).

J.J. Corrigan, 'The effect of vitamin E on warfarin-induced vitamin K deficiency' (1982) *A NY Acad Sci* 393:361-8.

E.J. Crary, G. Smyrna, M. McCarty, 'The potential clinical applications for high dose nutritional antioxidants' (1984) *Medical Hypotheses* 13:77-98.

W. Dalton, 'Massive doses of vitamin C in the treatment of viral disease' (Aug 1962)*J Indiana State Med Assn* 55:1151-4.

J.W. Dickerson, 'Vitamins and trace elements in the seriously ill patient' (1981) Acta Chir Scand 507: suppl.144-50.

J.R. Di Palma, D.M. Ritchie, 'Vitamin toxicity' (1977) Ann Rev Pharmacol Toxicol 17:133-48.

T.M. Florence, 'Cancer and ageing — the free radical connection' (1983) Chemistry in Australia, vol.50, no.6.

C. Fossati, 'Adverse reactions to vitamins' (1981) Clin Ther 99:643-51.

A.R. Gaby, 'The safe use of vitamin B6' (1990) J Nutr Med 1:153-9.

R. Goodhart, M. Shiels, Modern Nutrition in Health and Disease (Lea & Febiger, Philadelphia, 1980).

R.L. Gross et al, 'The role of nutrition in immunologic function' (1980) Physiology Review 60: no.1:188-302.

H.E. Harrison, 'Effects of nutrient toxicities in animals and man: vitamin D' in M. Rechcigl Jr (ed), CRC Handbook Series in Nutrition and Food (CRC Press, West Palm Beach, 1978, Section E: nutritional disorders, vol.1, pp.87-90).

K.C. Hayes, M.D. Hegsted, Toxicity of vitamins. Toxicants occurring naturally in foods (National Academy of Sciences, Washington, 1973).

V. Herbert, 'Megaloblastic anemia' (1963) N Engl J Med 268:201-3.

D. Hornig, U. Moser, 'The safety of high vitamin C intake in man' in J.N. Counsell and D.H. Hornig (eds) Vitamin C (Applied Science Publishers, 1981, pp.225-48).

D. Hornig, 'Ascorbic Acid — Vitamin C' in Counsell and Hornig, The Safety of High Vitamin C Intakes (Applied Science Publisher, pp.245).

Y. Itokawa, 'Effect of nutrient toxicities in animals and man: thiamine' in M. Rechigl jr (ed) CRC Handbooks Series in Nutrition and Food (CRC Press, West Palm Beach, 1978, pp.3 23, Section E: Nutritional disorders, vol. 1, Effect of nutrient excesses and toxicities in animals and man).

H. Kirchmair, B. Kirsch, 'Treatment of epidemic hepatitis in childhood with high doses of ascrobic acid' (1957) Medizinische Monathschrift 11:353-57.

F.R. Klenner, 'Massive doses of vitamin C and virus diseases' (1951) J Southern Med and Surgery 103:101-7.

F.R. Klenner, 'The treatment of poliomyelitis and other virus diseases with vitamin C' (July 1949) J Southern Med and Surgery 209-14.

R.P. Knott et al., 'Toxicity of pantothen' (1957) Proc Soc Exp Bio Med 95:340-1.

S. Lewin, Vitamin C, It's Molecular Biology and Medical Potential (New York Academic Press, 1976, 131-73).

J. Marks, A Guide to Vitamins: Their Role in Health and Disease (1975, MTP Press, Lancaster).

A. Mitwalli et al, 'Safety of intermediate doses of pyridoxine' (1984) Can Med Assoc 131-14.

F. Morishige, A. Murata, 'Vitamin C for prophylaxis of viral hepatitis B in transfused patients' (1978) J Intern Academy of Prev Med 5:54-58.

L.R. Mosher, 'Nicotinic acid side effects and toxicity: a review' (1970) Am J Psych 1290-96.

A. Murata, 'Viricidal activity of vitamin C: Vitamin C for prev and treatment of viral diseases.' Proceedings of the 1st Intersessional Congress of the International Association of the Microbiological Society (Tokyo University Press, 1975, pp.432-42) reported in E. Cheraskin et al, The Vitamin C Connection (Thorsens, 1983, pp.48-9).

National Research Council, Food and Nutrition Board Recommended Dietary Allowances (National Academy of Sciences, Washington, 1980, 9th rev. ed).

J.M. Paez de Latorre, 'The use of ascorbic acid in measles' (1945) Archivas Argentinos de Pediatra 24:225-6.

W.O. Pardue, 'Severe liver dysfunction during nicotinic acid therapy' (1961) J Am Med Ass 175:137-8.

W.B. Parsons jr, 'Activation of peptic ulcer by nicotinic acid report of five cases' (1960) J Am Med Ass 173:1466-70.

G. Reccuglia et al, 'Absorption and excretion of cyanocobalamine after oral administration of a large dose in various conditions' (1969) Acta Haematol 42:1-7.

E.H. Reynolds, 'Anticonvulsants, folic acid and epilepsy' (1973) Lancet 1:1376-78.

K.S. Roth, 'Biotin in clinical medicine. Review' (1981) Am J Clin Nutr 34:1967-74.

H. Schaumburg et al, 'Sensory neuropathy from pyridoxine abuse' (1983) N Engl J Med 311:986-7.

A. Shenkin, 'Additives in parenteral nutrition' (1981) Acta Chir Scand 507:suppl., pp.350-55.

I. Stone, The Healing Factor, Vitamin C Against Disease (Grosset and Dunlap, 1972, pp.70-89).

O. Truss, 'The role of candida albicans in human illness' (1981) J Ortho Psych vol.10, no.4:228-38.

P.C. Wilson, 'The effect of folic acid on the intestinal absorption of zinc'(1983) Clin Res 31:A760.

Chapter 8

I.Z. Beitins, A. Barkan, A. Kiblanski et al, 'Hormonal responses to short term fasting in post menopausal women' (1985) *J Clin Metab* 60:1120-6.

T.A. Brown, M.W. Russel, J. Mestecky, 'Elimination of intestinally absorbed antigen into the bile by IgA' (1984) *J Immunol* 132:780-2.

D.P. Burkitt, A.R.P. Walker, N.S. Painter, 'Effects of dietary fibre on stools and transit times and its role in the causation of disease' (1972) *Lancet* II:1408-12.

H.M. Cantor, A. Dumont, 'Hepatic suppression of sensitization to antigen absorbed into the portal system' (1967) *Nature* 215:744-5.

J.H. Cummings, 'Germentation in the human large intestine: Evidence and implications for health' (1983) *Lancet* 1:1208-8.

M.A. Eastman, J.R. Kirkpatrick, W.D. Mitchell et at, 'Effects of dietary supplements of wheat bran and cellulose on feces and bowel function' (1973) *Br Med J* 4:392-4.

J. Egger, C.M. Carter, J. Wilson et al, 'Is migraine food allergy?' (1983) *Lancet* II:865-9.

J. Finne, M. Leinonen, P.H. Makela, 'Antigenic similarities between brain components and bacteria causing meningitis' (1983) *Lancet* II:355-7.

B.A. Friend, K.M. Shahani, 'Nutritional and therapeutic aspects of lactobacili' (1984) *J App Nutr* 36:125-36.

P.J. Gallagher, N.J. Goulding, M.J. Gibney et al, 'Acute and chronic immunological response to dietary antigen' (1983) *Gut* 24:831-5.

W.A. Hemmings, 'The entry into the brain of large molecules derived from dietary protein' (1978) *Proc R Soc London Br* 200:175-92.

E.C. Hughes, L. Oettinger, F. Johnson, G.H. Gorttschalk, 'Case report: A clinically defined diet in diagnosis and management of food sensitivity in minimal brain dysfunction' (1979) *Ann Allergy* 42:174-6.

M. Imamura, T. Tung, 'A trial of fasting cure for PCB poisoned patients in Taiwan' (1984) *Am J Ind Med* 5:147-53.

T. Lawlor, D.G. Wells, 'Metabolic hazards of fasting' (1969) *Am J Clin Nutr* 22:8:1142-9.

H. Lithell, A. Bruce, I.B. Gustafsson, 'A fasting and vegetarian treatment trial on chronic inflammatory disorders' (1983) *Acta Derm Venerol (Stockh)* 63:397-403.

T. Nolan, 'The role of endotoxin in liver injury' (1975) *Gastroenterol* 69:1346-56.

R. Paganelli, R.J. Levinsky, D.J. Atherton, 'Detection of specific antigen within circulating immune complexes. Validation of the assay and its application to food antigen antibody complexes formed in healthy and food-allergic subjects' (1981) *Clin Exp Immunol* 46:44-53.

W.J. Rea, D.W. Peters, R.E. Smiley et al, 'Recurrent environmentally triggered thrombophlebitis. A five-year follow-up' (1981) *Ann Allergy* 47:338-44.

M.W. Russel, T.A. Brown, J.L. Claflin et al, 'Immunoglobulin A-mediated hepatobiliary transjport constitutes a natural pathway for disposing of bacterial antigens' (1983) *Infect Immunity* 42:1041-8.

N. Shah, T. Atallah, R.R. Mahoney, P.L. Pellett, 'Effect of dietary fibre components on fecal nitrogen excretion and protein utilization' (1982) *J Nutr* 112:658-66.

K.M. Shahani, Ad. Ayebo, 'Role of dietary lactobacilli in gastrointestinal microecology' (1980) *Am J Clin Nutr* 33:2448.

R.A. Shakman, 'Nutritional influences on the toxicity of environmental pollutants. A review' (1974) *Arch Env Health* 28:105-33.

L. Skoldstam, F.D. Lindstrom, B. Lindblom, 'Impaired con. A suppresor cell activity in patients with rheumatoid arthritis shows normalization during fasting' (1983) *Scand J Rheumatol* 12:4:369-73.

K. Stephansson, M.E. Dieperink, D.P. Richman et al, 'Sharing of antigenic determinants between the nicotinic acetylcholine receptor and proteins in Escherichia coli, Proteus vulgaris and Klebsiella pneumoniae' (1985) *N Eng J Med* 312:221-5.

T. Sundquist, F. Lindstrom, K. Magnusson, L. Skoldstam, 'Influence of fasting on intestinal permeability and disease activity in patients with rheumatoid arthritis shows normalization during fasting' (1982) *Scand J Rheumatol* 11:33-8.

J. Suzuki, Y. Yamauchi, M. Horikawa, S. Yamagata, 'Fasting therapy for psychosomatic disease with special reference to its indications and therapeutic mechanism' (1976) *Tohoku J Exp Med* 118(Suppl):245-59.

D.R. Triger, M.H. Alp, R. Wright, 'Bacterial and dietary antibodies in liver disease' (1972) *Lancet* 1:60-63.

A.M. Uden, L. Trang, N. Venizelos, J. Palmblad, 'Neutrophil function and clinical performances after total fasting in patients with rheumtoid arthritis' (1983) *Ann Rheum Dis* 42:45-51.

W.A. Walker, K.J. Isselbacher, 'Uptake and transport of macromolecules by the intestine: possible role in clinical disorders' (1974) *Gastroenterol* 66:987-92.

E.J. Wing, R.T. Stanko, A. Winnkelstein, S.A. Adibi, 'Fasting enhanced immune effector mechanism in obese patients' (1983) *Am J Med* 75:91-6.

C. Zioudrov, R.A. Streaty, W.A. Klee, 'Opioid peptides derived from food proteins' (1979) *J Biol Chem* 254:2446-9.

Chapter 9

R. Ader (ed), *Psychoneuroimmunology* (New York Academic Press, 1981).

G.H.B. Baker, D. Brewerton, 'Rheumatoid arthritis — a psychiatric assessment' (1981), *Br Med J*, 2014-282.

R.W. Bartrop, P. Luckhurst, L. Lazarus, L.G. Kiloh, R. Penny, 'Depressed lymphocyte function after bereavement' (1977) *Lancet*, 834-36.

S. Greer et al, 'Psychological response to breast cancer: effect on outcome' (1979) *Lancet* II:785-7.

J.B. Jemmot, 'Academic stress, power motivation and decrease in secretion rate of secretory immunoglobulin A' (1983) *Lancet* 1400-9.

S.V. Kasl et al, 'Psychosocial risk factors in the development of infectious mononucleosis' (1979) *Psychosom Med* 41:445-65.

Z. Kronfol et al, 'Impaired lymphocyte function in depressive illness' (1983) *Life Science* 33:241-7.

R.J. Meyer, R. Haggerty, 'Streptococcal infections in families: factors alerting individual susceptibility' (1962) *Pediatrics* 29:539-49.

S.J. Schliefer, S.E. Keller, M. Camerino, J.C. Thornton, M. Stein, 'Suppression of lymphocyte stimulation following bereavement' (1983) *JAMA* 250: 374-77.

R.B. Shekelle et al, 'Psychological depression and 17 year risk of death from cancer' (1981) *Psychosom Med* 43:117 256.

M. Werbach, *Nutritional Influences in Illness* (Third Line Press, California, 1987).

Chapter 10

M. Botez, S. Young, J. Bachevalier, S. Gauthier, 'Effect of folic acid and vitamin B12 deficiencies on 5 hydroxyindoleacetic acid in human cerebrospinal fluid' (1982) *Ann Neurol* 12:479-84.

D. Kripke, S. Risch, D. Janowsky, 'Bright white light alleviates depression' (1983), *Psychiat Res* 10:105-12.

A. Lewy, T. Wehr, F. Goodwin et al, 'Manic-depressive patients may be supersensitive to light' (1981) *Lancet* 1:383-4.

M. Peel, 'Rehabilitation in postviral syndrome' (1988) *J Soc Occup Med* 38:44-5.

N. Rosenthal, D. Sack, C. Carpenter et al, 'Antidepressant effects of light in seasonal affective disorders' (1985) *Am J Psychiat* 142:163-70.

N. Rosenthal, D. Sack, C. Gillin et al, 'Seasonal affective disorder: a description of the syndrome and preliminary findings with light treatment' (1984) *Arch Gen Psychiat* 41:72-80.

L. Wetterberg, 'The relationship between the pineal gland and the pituitary-adrenal axis in health, endocrine and psychiatric conditions' (1983) *Psychoneuroendocrinology* 8:75-80.

Glossary

Affirmations: Short positive statements that can be repeated to oneself as an aid to changing beliefs and/or undesirable feelings.
Aldrin: A highly toxic insecticide containing chlorine.
Allergens: Molecules that cause allergy, e.g. pollen grains, egg protein, house dust.
Antioxidants: Naturally occurring substances that neutralise the harmful effects of oxidising chemical reactions, e.g. vitamins C and E are naturally occurring antioxidants.
Antibody: A protein molecule produced by the immune system which can attach itself to a bacteria or virus and inactivate it. Some antibodies combine with allergens to produce allergic reactions. Hence antibodies may play a beneficial or harmful role in body functions.
Anticoagulant: A substance that stops the blood from clotting in the arteries and veins.
Antigen: Any foreign substance which when placed in the body's tissues stimulates the production of antibodies by the immune system.
Antihistamines: Usually drugs which neutralise or inhibit the effect of histamine in the body. Histamine is a chemical produced by the immune system during an allergic reaction. Antihistamines are therefore mainly used in the treatment of allergic disorders, e.g. hay fever. Naturally occurring antihistamines include vitamin C and bioflavonoids.
Anti-depressants: A class of drugs or naturally occurring substances used for elevating the mood in people suffering from depression. For example, tricyclic anti-depressants are drugs, tryptophan is a naturally occurring anti-depressant.
Atopic: The tendency within some families towards allergic diseases.
Auto-oxidation: Oxidation of the tissues with subsequent damage; due to abnormalities in the body's metabolism and a lack of suitably active antioxidant chemicals.
Auto-antibodies: Antibodies produced by the immune system that attack the body's own tissues and cells. For example, in rheumatoid arthritis the patient's own antibodies attack and destroy the joint tissues.
Auto-immune disease: A disease in which the body's own immune system produces antibodies and other substances which attack and destroy tissues and organs.
Beta blockers: A drug that blocks the effect of adrenalin in the nervous system and heart; used in treating angina and blood pressure.
Brain fag: A term used to describe extreme mental fatigue or exhaustion; probably the result of the nervous system's hypersensitivity reaction to some foods and/or chemicals.

Carcinogen: Any substance which tends to produce cancer in a living organism.
Central nervous system: Consists of the brain and the spinal cord which is nervous tissue extending from the brain down to the base of the spine.
Cerebro-spinal fluid: The fluid that bathes the brain and spinal cord and acts as a shock absorber to protect these delicate organs.
CFS: An abbreviation for the chronic fatigue syndrome (also chemical food sensitivity).
Chelation therapy: A form of therapy in which a medicine is given that binds to toxins or heavy metals in the body to make these noxious substances soluble in the blood so that they can be filtered out by the kidneys and excreted in the urine.
Corticosteroids: Hormones secreted by a small gland on top of the kidneys; commonly called cortisone.
Cortisol: One of the corticosteroid hormones secreted by the adrenal glands.
Cyclic AMP: A compound in cell membranes which activates enzymes within the body's cells; stimulated by hormones.
Depression — psychotic: A severe form of mental depression which includes the risk of suicide; requires psychiatric intervention and usually hospitalisation.
Depression — endogenous: A form of depression caused by internal factors — possibly dietary, food allergies, vitamin deficiencies. Exogenous depression is caused by some external factor such as the loss of a loved one.
Depression — manic: A severe mental disorder characterised by cyclical periods of mental over-excitation followed by depression.
Dieldrin: A highly toxic insecticide containing chlorine.
Double blind trials: A medical experiment in which a drug being tested is given to one group of individuals and a placebo (inactive substance) is given to another group of patients. Neither the treating doctors nor the patients know which is receiving the active or the inactive substance, hence the term double bind. At the end of the trial an independent worker decodes the information. In this way any psychological benefits gained from treatment are applied equally to both groups and any difference in outcome of treatment can be assumed to be solely due to the active drug.
Dysplasia: An abnormal development of cell structure and may be a precursor to a cancerous cell.
EB virus: The Epstein-Barr virus which is responsible for a chronic glandular fever-like syndrome.
ECG: Abbreviation for electrocardiogram which is the measurement of the heart's electrical activity by means of electrodes placed on the chest wall.
Eczema: A chronic inflammatory disorder of the skin due to allergies and nutritional deficiencies. The skin generally breaks down and can be very dry and scaly or it may weep with fluid; can be extremely itchy and uncomfortable.
EEC: Abbreviation for electroencephalogram and is a measurement of the brain's electrical activity by placing electrodes over the skull and measuring electrical impulses with a very sensitive graph machine.
Enzyme: A protein which is capable of increasing chemical reactions in living cells to very fast rates without actually changing itself. Enzymes are involved in every metabolic reaction in the body. Without enzymes, biological reactions would be so slow that life would not be possible.
Free radical: A highly reactive molecule which is electrically unbalanced and can cause untold damage to the body's cell membranes, proteins and genes. They are probably responsible for most degenerative diseases and possibly even cancer and the ageing process.
Genetics: The science of heredity which deals with the differences and resemblances

of living things and their inherited characteristics.
Holistic: Refers to the practice of medicine in which the whole individual is considered as a part of the total environment and that physical, psychological and spiritual factors contribute to health and disease.
Homeopathy: The science of treating diseases using drugs given in minute doses which produce in a healthy person symptoms similar to those of the disease the individual is suffering. For example, onions cause watering of the eyes and irritation in the nose — symptoms which mimic hay fever — so minute doses of onion extract can be used to treat the symptoms of hay fever.
Hypoglycaemia: Refers to low blood sugar (glucose). It is the opposite to diabetes in which there is a raised blood sugar due to a lack of insulin. Hypoglycaemia is the body's response to stress and a diet high in refined carbohydrates including sugar, white flour products and alcohol. Following a high intake of these substances, the body's reaction is to lower the blood sugar as quickly as possible and in doing so sometimes overshoots the normal lower limit resulting in sudden drops of blood sugar to very low levels. This can have disastrous effects on the nervous system and the immune system causing a wide range of symptoms.
I.U.: Abbreviation for international units, a measure of the activity of some vitamins; for example, vitamins A and E are measured in international units.
Iatrogenic disease: A disease caused or produced by the diagnosis or the treatment given by a medical doctor. For example, a bleeding duodenal ulcer caused by an anti-arthritis drug would be an iatrogenic disease. Two in five hospital beds are occupied by patients suffering iatrogenic diseases.
Immune system: The body's defence system against invasion by foreign substances including bacteria, viruses, foreign proteins and even such things as dusts and moulds. It consists of immune cells and antibodies. The antibodies bind on to the foreign invaders and present the invader to immune cells which then engulf and destroy the foreign substance with enzymes and free radicals.
Immuno-suppressive agent: A drug, chemical or even a hormone with actions that cause the suppression of the white blood cells of the immune system or the suppression of their ability to produce antibodies. As a consequence of immuno suppression, diseases such as infections, inflammations, auto immune diseases, lymphoma and cancer may result. Immuno suppressive agents include drugs, cortisone and most of the heavy metals and chemicals present in the environment.
Lactobacillus: A family of bacteria that can break down milk sugar called lactose to lactic acid. These bacteria are healthy bacteria that are used to make yoghurt and other soured milks. Lactobacilli live in the healthy vagina and bowel. Antibiotics kill lactobacilli and permit the overgrowth of undesirable micro-organisms in these organs. The use of lactobacilli in powder form can normalise the internal environment of the bowel and vagina.
Lipid: Another word for fat which include animal fats and oils. They all have a greasy feel and are insoluble in water. Lipids are very sensitive to many synthetic chemicals and because lipids make up the body's cell membranes, their protection is extremely important.
Lipoprotein: A compound consisting of both a lipid and a protein. For example, cholesterol is usually complexed with protein in the blood plasma.
Lymphocyte: A specialised white blood cell. May secrete antibodies, immune chemicals such as interferon or it may become super-specialised and act as a natural killer cell for the destruction of cancer cells in the body.
Lysosomes: Minute granules present inside living cells. They contain many enzymes which are responsible for the destruction of invading bacteria and viruses.
Macro-nutrients: Nutrients in the diet that form the bulk of the food; include

proteins, fats, carbohydrates and fibre.
Metabolism: The sum of all the chemical changes in a living cell in which food is incorporated into the cell structure and by which other food is broken down into simpler substances with the exchange of energy for cell function to continue.
Metabolites: The end product of metabolism and include organic acids, aldehydes, carbon dioxide and water; these must leave the living cell to be excreted from the body.
Micro-nutrients: Nutrients required in very small amounts but essential for health and the prevention of disease. Examples include vitamins, minerals and trace elements such as zinc and selenium.
Mitochondria: Minute granules present in living cells that are regarded as being responsible for the production of energy from food and oxygen. Mitochondria contain genetic material that may be responsible for the ageing process. Disturbances in mitochondrial function probably play a role in the chronic fatigue syndrome.
Myalgia: Muscle pain.
Narcolepsy: A condition characterised by the uncontrollable desire for sleep at almost any time.
Neuropsychological: Symptoms referrable to the central nervous system and the mind. For example, headaches are neurological disorders and anxiety states are regarded as psychological disorders. A person suffering from both headaches and anxiety could be described as suffering from neuropsychological symptoms.
Neuropsychologist: A trained professional who specialises in the study of neurological and psychological disease.
Neurosis: An emotional disorder whereby feelings of tension, anxiety, obsessional thoughts and physical complaints without evidence of organic disease predominate within the personality of the individual. With better understanding of allergy, chemical sensitivity and body chemistry, neuroses are no longer regarded as purely emotional by medical specialists in the field of nutritional medicine.
Neurotransmitter: A naturally occurring chemical in the brain that travels from one nerve cell to another. Neurotransmitters are therefore the nervous system's communications agents. All of these neurotransmitters are derived from the food we eat and their activity can be influenced by dietary changes.
Nightshade family: A group of plants belonging to the Solanacea family which include potatoes, tomatoes, eggplant, capsicum and tobacco.
Nitrosamines: Cancer causing chemicals that are formed in the human gastrointestinal tract from nitrites in the diet. The nitrites are obtained from artificial fertilisers in the foods we eat. The formation of nitrosamines can be prevented by using supplements of vitamin C in the diet.
NK cells: Known as natural killer cells and are specialised white blood cells involved in the destruction of cancers.
Opium-based pain killers: A group of chemicals related to opium and include morphine, codeine and pethidine; they are addictive and their use is reserved for severe pain.
Organochlorine: An organic molecule containing chlorine atoms in its structure. Organochlorine chemicals are commonly used as pesticides and herbicides. They are very reactive, poisonous and potentially carcinogenic.
Pathogenic: Refers to the ability to produce disease in a living thing.
Periconceptual: Refers to the period of time just prior to, during and after conception. Periconceptual nutrition involves the provision of ideal nutrition to both the male and female prior to conception.
Perinatal: Pertaining to the period closest to the time of birth.

Phorbol esters: A family of pesticides.

Prostaglandins: A family of hormone-like substances derived from essential fatty acids in the diet. For example, certain fish oils and evening primrose oil contain essential fatty acids that are converted in the body to hormone-like molecules that have widespread effects on most cell tissues in the body.

RDA: Abbreviation for recommended daily allowance. This is the allowance of nutrients recommended by most government authorities. The levels recommended are intended to prevent deficiency disease in the majority of the population. However, they do not refer to levels of micro-nutrients for the promotion of optimum good health.

Sedatives: May be a drug or a naturally occurring substance that has a relaxing or sedating effect on the central nervous system. For example, the drug Valium is a synthetic sedative whereas the herb passionflower is a natural sedative.

The 'sick building' syndrome: Refers to a collection of symptoms including fatigue, headaches, sore eyes, stuffy noise, sore throat, muscle aches and pains and other less specific symptoms that occur in some people when confined to closed modern buildings. The high concentrations of synthetic chemicals in modern office buildings is probably the reason for most of the symptoms in this syndrome. However, poor quality air, unnatural lighting and the production of negative ions from electronic equipment are also incriminated.

Solvents: Chemical solvents are highly reactive fluids used in industry and the home for dissolving substances, for example in printing and cleaning.

Spina bifida: A congenital abnormality in the development of the spine in which the spinal cord may be exposed to the external environment. Spina bifida has been shown to be prevented by the prescription of vitamin B-complex prior to and during pregnancy.

Symptomatic treatment: Treatment aimed at relieving symptoms. For example, the use of a pain killer to relieve migraine. This compares with a more favourable and scientific approach now adopted by many doctors and natural therapists in which the causes of the migraine are sought and, if possible, removed.

Synergism: Refers to the working together of substances. For example, the combined action of two medications or nutrients is greater than the sum of the individual activities. One substance increases the effectiveness of the other and vice versa. We can have positive synergism as in the use of a vitamin and mineral together in the diet to give greater benefit than either used alone, or negative synergism in which two synthetic chemicals can do a certain amount of harm but when combined the damage is even greater.

Tinnitus: A ringing in the ears that can become so severe as to cause severe depression. May be due to chemical sensitivities and/or deficiencies of some nutrients.

Tranquilliser: May be a synthetic chemical drug or a naturally occurring substance such as the herb valerian.

T-cells: Special white blood cells of the immune system.

T-lymphocyte: Identical to a T-cell.

Xenobiotic: A xenobiotic chemical is a synthetic chemical usually of high toxicity.

Index

A

abdominal pains, 13, 14, 151, 160, 169, 176
affirmations, 189-190, 204
Agent Orange, 99, 104
AIDS, 61, 64, 68, 184
Alaskan Dental Association, 44, 48
alcohol, 2, 10, 17, 20, 24, 25, 27, 30-31, 58-59, 61, 72-73, 81, 108, 114-115, 136, 144, 146, 155, 163-164, 179, 194
allergies, 2, 4-5, 25, 31, 52, 70, 77, 89, 106, 108, 114, 149, 153, 157, 161, 165
aluminium, 34-35, 77, 176
amalgam, 40, 42-45, 47, 77, 176, 203, 214
 see also dental fillings
 symptoms of incompatibility, 49
amino acids, 20, 122, 145, 150, 168, 176, 204
anaemia, 1, 120, 124-125, 134
anger, 14, 54
antibiotics, 8, 32, 62, 71-73, 144, 164, 166
antihistamines, 24, 30
anti-inflamatory, 30, 85, 92, 155
anti-oxidants, 83-85, 89, 91-93, 96, 130, 132, 143, 144, 155, 156, 217
appetite, 11, 13 19, 20
arsenic, 34-35, 42, 77, 136, 174, 176
arthritis, 2, 24, 27, 31, 64, 70, 107, 108, 110, 116, 146, 151, 153-154, 160, 217
asthma, 24, 27, 99, 108, 113-114, 122, 151, 153, 217
Australia, 42, 48, 78, 94
auto-immune disease, 2, 53, 64, 134

B

back pain, 4, 14
beta-blockers, 24, 77-78, 155
biotin, 123, 128
bowel, 143-144, 152, 155, 160-163, 164, 166-167, 170-172, 174, 177-178, 180, 203
breast tenderness, 3, 13

C

cadmium, 34-35, 38, 42, 77
calcium, 38, 118, 123, 140
Californian Dental Association, 46
Canada, 48, 97
cancer, 2, 9, 12, 27, 33, 56, 64, 68, 70, 90-91, 93, 104, 132, 133-134, 136, 151, 154, 160, 165, 170, 184, 217
candida, 9, 34, 54, 56, 59, 71, 72, 73, 77, 143, 160, 165-166, 167
 see also thrush
chelation, 90, 143
chelation therapy, 175-177, 214
chicken pox, 34, 60, 134-135
chromium, 30, 38, 70, 123-124, 129, 174
chronic fatigue syndrome, 1
 causes of, 34
 controversial aspects, 10
 definition of, 1
 symptoms of, 5
 history of, 8
 social consequences, 10
 triggers of, 8-9
 diagnostic criteria, 67
colon, 159, 160, 169
colon therapy, 158-159, 172
contraceptive pill, 24, 72, 155
copper, 34, 38, 42, 123, 130

cortisone, 30, 64, 72, 122, 155
coxsackie virus, 33, 34
cytomegalovirus, 33, 34, 56, 60, 61, 65

D
DDD, 78, 82, 98
DDE, 78, 82, 98
DDT, 78, 82, 98, 153
dementia, 24, 96, 97
dental fillings, 40, 42–43, 47, 49, 77, 176
 removal of, 49, 50–52, 203, 215
dentists, 45
depression, 2, 3, 6, 11
 causes of, 15,
 CFS associated, 11
 definition of, 11
 diagnosis of, 19
 effects of, 18
 manic, 7, 27
 masked, 21
 mild, 11, 22
 premenstrual, 13
 psychotic, 7
 relief from, 27
 severe, 12, 17, 21, 23, 25
 symptoms of, 22
 types of, 22
detoxification, 82, 100, 121, 132, 135–136, 142–145, 147, 150, 156–158, 162, 172–174
diabetes, 2, 24, 27, 30, 33, 53, 70, 151–152, 154, 160, 179, 217
dairy products, 26, 106–108, 114, 115, 152, 157, 163, 168, 170
dieldrin, 78, 98
dioxin, 99

E
eczema, 27, 106, 113–114, 116, 153
electric shock treatment, 14, 15
electromagnetic
 fields, 54, 105
 pollution, 104, 143
Epstein-Barr virus, 33–34, 56–60, 63–65
essential fatty acids, 123, 130, 145, 156, 174
exercise, 147, 152, 161, 172, 196, 208, 209, 210, 211, 212

F
fasting, 78, 87, 90, 115, 147, 148, 149, 150, 151, 152, 160,
fatigue, 1
 definition of, 1
 treatment summary, 195
folic acid, 46, 62, 116, 118, 123, 127, 165
free radicals, 79, 84–86, 88–89, 92, 93, 130–132, 155, 173
free radical disease, 81, 83, 87, 144
 definition of, 81
fruits, cleansing, 156

G
German measles, 34, 134
glandular fever, 6, 26, 34, 56, 61–63, 134–135

H
headaches, 7, 11, 13, 20, 99, 110, 115, 152, 160
heart disease, 2, 9, 24, 27, 30, 33, 77, 113, 134, 151, 154, 160, 217
heat therapies, 206–208
hepatitis, 26, 63, 134, 170
heavy metals, 34, 135, 143, 149, 174
herbicides, 76–77, 93, 95, 97, 143, 149, 152, 161
herbs, 60, 73, 116, 138, 144–147, 159, 203
herpes, 56, 60, 65, 134

I
Icelandic disease, 6
immune system, 8–9, 35, 53, 61, 72, 96, 107, 118, 120, 144, 161–162, 194
inflammatory disorders, 31, 64, 70, 91, 146, 153, 154
interferon, 68–70
irritable bowel syndrome, 4, 48, 73, 111, 119, 151, 153, 160
iron, 38, 123

K
kidneys, 143–144, 155, 176, 214
kidney disease, 31

L
lactobacillus, 73, 152, 163, 165–171
lead, 34–35, 42, 77–78, 135–136, 143, 174–176

symptoms of poisoning, 36
  airborne, 37
  contamination sources, 38
leukaemia, 31, 132, 134
liver, 144–146, 155, 161–162, 172, 179
liver disease 31, 170–171
lymphatic function, 144, 146–147

M
magnesium, 3, 118, 123
massage, 146–147
meals, 197
  timing of, 200
measles, 34, 65
meditation, 184–192
menopause, 31
mercury, 34–35, 40, 42–43, 50, 78, 135–136, 143, 174–176, 215
  excretion of, 47
  toxicity, 39, 52
  sensitivity, 39
  symptoms of poisoning, 40
migraine headaches, 4, 51, 106, 108, 110, 114, 119, 151, 152, 160
minerals, 20, 31, 116, 118, 122, 140
moods, 15, 18, 27, 68, 70, 97, 117
multiple sclerosis, 24, 31, 43, 53, 64
mumps, 34
myalgic encephalomyelitis (ME), 6–7, 14
  history of, 8

N
nervous system, 7, 9, 14, 20, 35–36, 41, 52, 54, 63, 68, 76, 96, 109, 118, 149, 161, 168, 171, 176, 179
niacin, 90, 123
nutritional supplements, 201–203

O
organochlorine, 78, 94
organophosphates, 98, 100
Orthomolecular Medical Association of Australia, 97
ozone, 103

P
PCBs, 99–100
Parkinson's disease, 24
penicillamine, 39, 50
periods, 13
pesticides, 76–77, 81, 93, 95–98, 100–101, 104, 143, 149, 152, 161
premenstrual syndrome, 3
premenstrual tension, 14
psoriasis, 153

R
relaxation, 181–182
respiratory disorders, 2, 99, 112
Roman Empire, 35–36
Ross River virus, 34
Royal Free Hospital disease, 6, 8

S
saunas, 144, 206–208
schizophrenia, 7, 18, 24, 27, 31, 149
seasonal affective disorder (SAD), 213
sex, 12, 18, 20, 21
'sick building' syndrome, 17, 31, 94
skin disorders, 4, 106, 108, 110, 114, 117, 119, 160, 166
sleep, 5, 12–13, 18, 20, 31, 69, 124, 155, 178, 185, 189
smog, 77–78, 104, 143
snacks, 196
spina bifida, 46, 93
stress, 2–3
  management, 4
stroke, 9, 154, 160, 217
suicide, 2, 10, 18, 21, 24, 25, 50–51, 104
sunlight, 213
Sweden, 49, 55
synergism, 95–96

T
teenagers, 6, 61
thiamine, 39, 122, 125, 140
  see also vitamin B1
thrush, 9, 34, 54, 59, 72, 160, 165–166
thyroid failure, 31
tiredness, 30
  causes of, 30
tobacco, 17, 26, 44, 114–115, 144, 155, 194, 196
trace elements, 20, 31
tranquillisers, 14, 24, 30

U
United States, 42–43, 48, 78, 94

V
vegetables, cleansing, 156

INDEX

vitamins, 20, 31, 38, 100, 116, 118, 122, 124, 137, 138
  A, 32, 83, 90, 123, 135, 138-139, 143
  B, 3, 117, 168
  B1, 38-39, 118, 122-123, 125, 135, 140
  B2, 118, 125
  B3, 90, 97-98, 118, 123, 126, 140
  B5, 123, 126
  B6, 118, 123, 126, 135, 138-139, 140
  B12, 46, 62, 116, 118, 120-124, 126, 135-136, 140, 165, 168
  B-complex, 30, 38, 46, 50, 62, 71, 98, 116, 124, 135, 137, 138, 140, 165, 168, 174-175, 194, 214
  C, 38, 50, 57, 62, 71, 82, 90, 92, 116-118, 123-124, 130-138, 140, 143-145, 156, 169, 172, 175-176, 194, 214, 217
  dependency, 15, 98,
  deficiencies, signs of, 124-127
  D, 138-139
  E, 90-92, 116, 130, 140, 173-174

K, 165, 168
recommended doses, 138-140

W
weight, 13, 19, 20-21, 77, 157, 200

X
xenobiotic
  overload or sensitivity, 34, 76
  chemicals, 71-72, 161
  transormation, 94

Y
yeast, 8-9, 54, 59, 71-73, 77, 160, 165-167, 171
yoga, 147, 152, 196, 208-209, 212
yuppie flu, 6

Z
zinc, 9, 19, 30, 38, 42, 50, 71, 97, 116-117, 118, 123-124, 128, 130, 137, 143, 174-175, 194, 198

Also in this series:

When Someone you Care for is Dying *by Norma Upson and Anna Potter*

Overcoming Pain *by Dr Leonard Rose*

Staying Rational in an Irrational World *by Dr Michael Bernard*

Mirrors of the Mind — The Creative Powers of Your Imagination *by Dr Leonard Rose with Peter Fitzgerald*